# FOODS
# FOR
# HEALTHY
# KIDS

BOOKS BY LENDON SMITH, M.D.

The Children's Doctor
The Encyclopedia of Baby and Child Care
New Wives' Tales
Improving Your Child's Behavior Chemistry
Feed Your Kids Right
Foods for Healthy Kids

# FOODS FOR HEALTHY KIDS

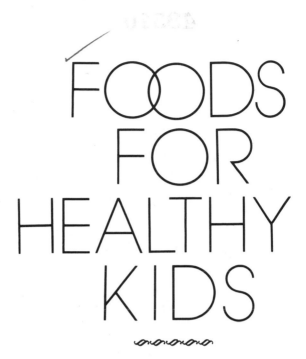

## Lendon Smith, M.D.

McGraw-Hill Book Company

New York   St. Louis   San Francisco
Toronto   Hamburg   Mexico

This book is not intended to replace the services of a physician. Any application of the recommendations set forth in the following pages is at the reader's discretion and sole risk.

LIBRARY OF CONGRESS CATALOGING IN PUBLICATION DATA

Smith, Lendon H., 1921–
Foods for healthy kids.
Includes index.
1. Children—Nutrition.  2. Children—Diseases—Nutritional aspects.  I. Title.
RJ206.S63    613.2'088054    81-2386
ISBN 0-07-058501-6    AACR2

Book design by Roberta Rezk.

I dedicate this book to my wife Julie, who has fed me well and provided a reason for hanging on so I could experience the pleasure of meeting my perfect grandchildren, Zachary, Gavin, Sirota, and Tage. It all shows what good genes and proper diet can produce. Love along the way helps also.

# Acknowledgments

A number of experts helped me with the recipes and text. They know the value of good food, simply and tastefully prepared. Healthy food does not have to taste like roots, blossoms, and bark. Sure, there is some honey dribbled around these pages, but only to get the sweet-lovers of the family to switch gradually to the good side.

Mary Ann Pickard has been a strong, helpful, without-which-nothing right arm. To meet a press deadline Mrs. Pickard put together the snacks that appear in the Foods for Restless Kids section to promote somnolence. She then took the foods one evening and tested them on a panel of experts— real live children. Only one recipe failed; it is not in this book.

Mrs. Pickard is married to a kind and well-fed dentist and has three young children. She is a nutritionist who learned from experience how to cook delicious whole foods without refined sugar or overmilled and devitalized grains. Her first immensely successful cookbook was *Feasting Naturally*, which has led thousands to a better life through good food without sacrificing taste, ease of preparation, or cost. *Feasting Naturally from Your Own Recipes* contains additional recipes and also helps the reader convert favorite recipes to better-tasting and more wholesome fare. She welcomes inquiries at P.O. Box 968, Harrison, Arkansas 72601.

Anastasia C. Condas is the mother of two teenagers and has teaching experience at all levels from nursery to graduate school. She has both a reading specialist and a learning disabilities credential and is currently the reading specialist at a California high school where she conducts a reading program that has been chosen one of three finalists for the California School Boards Association Golden Bell Award for 1980–1981.

Since she is the offspring of Greek immigrants, with a restaurateur for a father, good eating and wholesome food have always been a part of Mrs. Condas' life. Her past nine years of work with remedial students have also made her acutely aware of the effects of food on behavior and learning. Mrs. Condas is a founder and organizer of BEANS (Better Educational and Nutritional Standards), which effectively promotes local and state legislation and has helped raise the nutrition consciousness of parents and educators nationally. In conjunction with her work with BEANS she edited two recipe books, *Junk Food Alternative Requests* and *More Junk Food Alternatives,* as well as a how-to guide to eliminate junk food from the schools, *Dump the Junk.* (More information about BEANS and its activities is available by writing to Anastasia Condas, 17766 Hillside Court, Castro Valley, California 94546.)

Norma S. Upson lives in Oregon and has been invaluable in putting the recipes together, having tested and revised them with me a number of times. A freelance writer, Ms. Upson is also a columnist and lecturer. She is the author of *How to Survive as a Corporate Wife, The Crawfish Cookbook,* and *The Eggplant Cookbook.*

Kathy Mills lives in California and is the mother of three lively children who, along with many of the neighborhood children, act as her taste-testers. If children liked the recipes she invented, we used them in this book.

Myrtle Sherman is also a Californian with a master's degree in special education. She is a private consultant on curriculum in early childhood education, holds workshops in nutrition, and teaches child development and parenting classes. Mrs. Sherman routinely saw the relationship of diet and behavioral development as she reared and fed her six children and witnessed the improvement of foster children's health when they were fed in her home. Mrs. Sherman is also on the board of directors of the California State Task Force for Positive Parenting.

Linda Davis is an old friend from Chicago who works as a teacher and conducts nutritional workshops in suburban Chicago schools. Her message is clear and straight: If children don't eat good food the brain will not work well and good teaching will not be effective. Children must bring their brains to school.

Claire Berger is a resident of Colorado and wrote the *No Sugar, No Salt, No Additive* cookbook. She made solid contributions to the nourishing and tasty foods in this book.

My constant thanks to my assistant Peggy Moss, who has been at the beginning of all my writing. Given my deteriorating handwriting, I am amazed that she can read anything I scribble and even transcribe it into something better than what I originally wrote.

And special thanks go to Dr. David K. Shefrin, a naturopathic physician of Great Falls, Montana, who has been supportive and informative.

# Contents

# FOODS
# FOR
# HEALTHY
# KIDS

# Introduction

In my pediatric practice I see many children who simply "don't feel good." When they don't feel well, they are likely to become surly, demanding, hyperactive, or withdrawn. This antisocial behavior in turn stimulates the child's environment to respond negatively. If children are constantly told to "shut up," "sit down," or "get out," they are likely to develop a bad self-image. Thus psychological problems may develop as a result of neurobiochemical and nutritional factors.

We cannot live inside the bodies of our children and perceive what they perceive, but we can read their bodies for the clues that mean partial or outright physical slippage into some disease.

These deviations from normal well-being may be the result of genetic, pregnancy and delivery, or nutritional factors coupled with environmental stresses. Once symptoms appear we know the child is no longer able to screen out the debilitating stimuli. When the neocortex of the brain senses danger, it signals the pituitary, the adrenals, other organs, and the muscles to help handle the problem. If these organs are overstimulated and not replenished with rest and *adequate nutrition,* illness is the result. Asthma, migraine, hypertension, ulcers, hives, spastic colon, paranoia, and other murky problems can be traced to the interaction of stress and poor nutrition acting upon susceptible genes. Bacterial, viral, and fungal infections tell us that the body's immune systems are overstressed.

A child with a poorly functioning stimuli-filtering system might assume that a classroom is scary—too many sounds, too many movements. The child's response is to withdraw; he or she might shield his or her eyes, suck the thumb, and gently rock. Another overly sensitive child might run or talk or clown. Still another might start to wheeze.

They are asking for our help. One child may need calcium, one might be more comfortable with $B_6$, and pantothenic acid should help exhausted adrenal glands. Finally, they may all need a day off—or a different teacher.

Getting sick, having allergies, and developing a bad self-image are largely avoided by eating a nourishing diet and taking vitamin and mineral supplements. Children who are hyperactive, ticklish, who crave certain foods or sugar, are deep or light sleepers, have allergies, show Jekyll-and-Hyde behavior, and who need to rock, twist, suck, and wiggle can be helped with optimal nutrition. These symptoms and signs are *body clues* that suggest some system or organ is not functioning adequately because of faulty nutrition.

From birth on, children give us all sorts of clues to indicate that some trouble is ahead, sooner or later. Frequent colds, coughs, and respiratory phlegm alert us to the allergic child. Something can be done to avoid the nasty complications of ear, sinus, and bronchial infections. These early warning signs should alert the reasonably aware parent that there is a slippage from the ideal state of health, but chances are it is an easily reversible condition which should respond to a nutritional support system. You can wipe the child's nose, turn on the steam, and call the doctor. The doctor wants to help, so an antihistamine decongestant is prescribed. But the drug merely treats the phlegm.

In medical school we learned the pathophysiology of the disease process so we could more logically, skillfully, and swiftly treat the illness. But there was not one lecture or study about what initiated the fall from health.

The whole principle of our medical-school education was to make us superior diagnosticians. We were then expected to go with confidence and cure the world's ills. We were taught that there is an answer to every problem that comes into the office. If one missed a diagnosis, it meant one had slept through the appropriate lecture, but we had textbooks and could look up things if it got too tough. Once we had made the diagnosis, the medical or surgical treatment was easily initiated. The patient recovered, the parents were grateful, and the bill was paid. A nice clean system. For those patients in whom the diagnosis was in the gray area between palpable or visible pathology and psychoneurosis, we soon had tranquilizers, energizers, and pain-killers. For continuing complainers, we used the psychiatrist as the last resort. It was an admission of defeat that we could not find an organic answer. A psychiatric referral also meant that the parents had probably screwed up somehow. One could smell the guilt.

All this was neat and tidy. New patients came to me because they had been recommended by satisfied parents of patients; it was rewarding. And if we gave the drug companies enough time, we would have a specific, safe remedy for every condition known to afflict humans. Encouraged by this thought, we continued to prescribe their drugs so they would continue their research. If we helped them, they would eventually help us.

Yes, this is a neat and tidy system if the basic premise of medical practice is to diagnose and prescribe. But why did the patient get sick in the first place? Couldn't preventive medicine be practiced simultaneously? Why not start from the premise that if the body is operating optimally, it will not get sick?

All of us in practice soon became aware that some children (and adults) get sick all the time and some never get sick. Why the difference? Bad genes? Lack of care? Inadequate diet? Doctors are so busy diagnosing and treating, that they have no time to study these questions. A dentist said that the average person in our country has three cavities by age three years, fifteen cavities by adolescence, and is edentulous by the age of fifty. Does "average" mean "normal?"

In practice I learned not every stomachache is appendicitis. More often it's gas; most often it's pinworms (although one 2-A.M. screamer turned out to have a duodenal ulcer). After three decades I now realize that many of the medical principles we were taught as if etched in stone were advertising slogans or old wives' tales.

When I answer a parent's question I sometimes wonder just where the answer is really coming from. Is it filed next to clear immutables like "fires are hot" or is it in a little cloudy secluded area in which my mother and auntie dropped things such as "If you eat seeds, you get appendicitis," "You get tuberculosis from sleeping in closed rooms at night"? There is another area in my brain that has a collection of scientific "things." Many were "facts" when I learned them but have since been found to be half-truths or out-and-out lies (for example: the big thymus caused sudden infant death).

We were told to keep an open mind when we got our

MD degrees. I like the parting shot by the medical school dean to the newly matriculated students: "Gentlemen, I have some bad news. Half of what we taught you in the last four years is not true." Audible groaning. "The really distressing part of all this is we don't know which half."

I stumbled into the nutritional connection some years ago when a number of mothers of patients of mine told me that when they changed their diets, especially eliminating sugar and additives, their children were calmer, happier, and free from allergies and infections. I had trouble accepting that observation as a universal truism because it had not been taught to us in medical school.

But medical school had not helped me answer questions like "Why is my child sick all the time?" I found it embarrassing to say "Some kids are like that" or "Bad genes from the father's side." I needed better answers than the old cliché "He had this before? Well, he's got it again."

On reflection I realized that if hereditary factors are playing a role in susceptibility to sickness and odd behavior, the pathway from genes to the manifest disease has to have a biochemical connection. The genes are responsible for the enzymes that make the chemicals and hormones that run our bodies. Maybe these systems are not getting enough vitamins, amino acids, and minerals to make them run smoothly. Maybe some genetically poorly functioning enzyme system could do a better job if the nutrition were optimal. Accumulating evidence indicates that optimal nutrition will counteract the influence of debilitating genetic factors.

This book should provide parents with sufficient insight to detect the early warning signs that are the harbingers of big, scary diseases down the road. The body is throwing out clues to tell us that there is a slip from optimum health. The trick is to read the body's signs early enough, take nutritional action, and reverse the trend so the child does not *need* so much of the doctor's healing arts.

In *Foods For Healthy Kids* we emphasize diet and the use of foods in a prophylactic and therapeutic way. All of us could do better if we ate a more nourishing diet and took some supplements, but mainly avoided all sugars, processed foods, dairy fats and beef fat (low-fat cheese may be OK). We must persuade all food shoppers to follow this dictum: buy only nourishing foods. If sweets are in the house, they will be eaten. If there is diabetes, alcoholism, or obesity in the family genes, sugar in any form should be a major taboo.

We now know that some physical conditions and deviant behavior patterns suggest deficiencies of certain vitamins and minerals. We are suggesting that nutritional therapy be tried before or along with the doctor's therapies. Nothing is incompatible with these nutritional ideas except failure to try them. As Sara Sloan, head of Fulton County School System's Nutra Program (Atlanta, Georgia), says, "These nutritional ideas are not for everyone; only for those who wish to feel better."

What I hope to do is get some of the health care of children—and adults—back into the hands of parents and family. Loved ones and friends know each other well enough to be able to detect a deviation from the routine patterns; gait, cheek color, appetite, breath odor all combine into a constellation that says "Oops, he's going to be sick tomorrow."

Health is too important to leave it completely in the hands of the doctor. He can treat the symptoms once they become obviously diagnosable by stethoscope and microscope. We must explode the myth that cavities, allergies, sickness, headaches, and moodiness are inevitable. Most of us can live a comfortable life, be reasonably free of disease, and able to handle most of life's stresses if our bodies are properly nourished.

Those who have already established a pattern of sickness, allergy, hyperactivity, depression, or drug dependency should consult their doctor as well. As an example, if a child has had a few ear infections, cutting out milk and sugar and increasing calcium and vitamin C-bearing foods may not be adequate. He may need 1000 to 10,000 mg of vitamin C supplement per day for a month or two to recharge his depleted immune system. Then the optimum diet may suffice, but with special emphasis on the vitamin C and calcium recipes.

The recipes I have included in this book are for children (and adults) who wish to maintain good health. Each recipe is coded with a scorecard of its individual nutrients— protein, B vitamins, vitamin C—with stars next to each to rate the content: ★★★★ means tops, ★★★ good, ★★ fair, ★ trace.

These recipes will answer the harassed mother's cry, "What foods should my child eat? How do I get it into his stomach?" If the child (or spouse) believes it is inedible unless loaded with sugar, then honey, chemical sweeteners and fructose are—except to a jaded, already sugar-drenched palate—temporary crutches. The use of these products only serves to promote the idea that food must taste sweet. Some of the recipes in this book call for a sweetener, but they are just as delicious without it. Use the sweet substitutes at first if you wish, then gradually reduce them over a period of three months. In most families gradualism is easier than cold turkey.

The same applies to salt. Putting kelp or sea salt

in the salt cellar for those who salt everything before tasting it should help them gradually kick this bad habit.

Our Stone-Age bodies and intestinal tracts were specifically designed to chew, swallow, digest, absorb, and utilize the foods found on the earth. It follows that if a food has been processed, packaged, added to, milled, denatured, it is less than natural and will be digested with increasing difficulty. The vitamins and minerals needed for human utilization are neatly balanced in the foods Mother Nature hands us. If you have ever eaten a piece of white bread, then you are deprived to the extent that to metabolize the calories in that dough, your intestines and liver had to find the B vitamins and some minerals elsewhere in the body. It should have accompanied the food. We are all deprived.

To interpret most properly the lessons of Mother Nature, we should be eating 50 to 80 percent of our food in the raw or in a barely steamed state. Our mouths and guts are designed to digest large amounts of raw foods. Seeds, nuts, fruits, and raw vegetables should be our staples, and meat, cheese, fish, eggs, legumes, cereals, and breads should be used to add a little balance.

In these recipes we emphasize cooked things. We need recipes for cooked things. If we were optimally consistent with the philosophy of maximum nutrition, half the recipes would read something like this: Pick a fresh apple from a tree. Wash in soap and water or vinegar water. Eat and enjoy. (Chew and swallow seeds.)

These recipes should be used by everyone, child or adult, sick or well. They are just good nutrition. You and your child will feel better and act better with simple, nourishing food. If the body is provided with the proper nutrients, it usually restores itself. If symptoms persist, see your doctor. It is possible, however, that you or your child may be in such a nutritional hole that you will need some mega doses of some vitamins or some special counseling, nutritional or otherwise, to get your body working properly again.

If you are just beginning to introduce more fortified, nutritious foods to your child, start with a positive attitude. Don't apologize for the foods; a simple explanation that you are learning how to find better foods for the *whole family* will suffice. By all means, do not uphold a double standard: soft drinks and candy bars for you, cheese and orange juice for them! If they see you eating these foods, chances are very good that they will follow your example.

Help yourself and your children by eliminating all the undesirable sugared, packaged, and processed foods from your kitchen. If everything in the refrigerator is acceptable and your child has the freedom of choice, he will eat something healthful sooner or later.

Start out with tastes and dishes he is familiar with: taco salad (page 181), pizza (page 173), meat loaf (page 170), spaghetti (page 133). For breakfast, offer Super Sesame Oatmeal instead of the instant kind. Try baked eggs, too—many children enjoy eggs for breakfast, and these are especially quick and easy. Your own creativity will take over, and soon you'll be adapting and fortifying old favorites while you create new taste treats for your family.

# Reading 1 the Body

People living together are probably the most reliable observers of subtle changes of feeling, mood, expression, gait, odor, and sleep habits in each other. These changes represent the first shift away from biochemical equilibrium. Early minimal nutritional adjustment will usually get the body back to its optimal functioning.

The following levels of health are adapted from my book *Feed Your Kids Right*. These rather arbitrary divisions can help parents recognize slips from normal health in their children that could eventually lead to illness or behavioral problems. These clues and symptoms are readable in the body and are crying out for remediation. We need to understand what these clues mean and then help the body to heal itself by giving it all the nutriments it requires.

## Level I

This infant grows to adulthood free of illness, rashes, gas, headaches, fatigue, depression, insomnia. He* came from a stress-free, comfortable, full-term pregnancy and easy delivery. He laughs and smiles more than he cries and frowns. His hair and nails are glossy, not brittle, require a minimum of care, and his scalp is smooth and clean. His bowel movements have an acid odor with little or no putrid, nauseating smell. He's never constipated (well, hardly ever) nor does he have loose, sloppy, green BMs. He does not bruise easily, nor can one raise a wheal easily by scratching his skin. When he cries his nose runs clear; he breathes easily with no hyponasal twang to his voice. He sneezes, snores, and coughs rarely. No blood is noticed from his nose unless injured, and then it stops quickly.

He cuts teeth easily. He handles weather changes, teething, going to school, learning new skills, athletic exertion, and other stresses with a minimum of psychosomatic symptoms.

He is likely to come from a family that seems calm and accepting. There is little or no obesity, diabetes, allergy, alcoholism, schizophrenia, or depression in his family background.

He works up to his ability in school, is not easily distracted, learns to read easily, finishes assigned work, is usually compliant and easygoing. He makes friends easily and has a pleasant personality. He is adroit and coordinated. He is neither thin nor fat.

He has few extremes of emotional response—he cries or laughs appropriately. He enjoys doing things for others.

He sails through his developmental levels of physi-

---

* The word *he*, used in these examples and throughout this book, is of course the generic use—still a kind of communication shorthand—and almost always really means "he *or* she."

cal, psychological, and cognitive growth as if he had read the charts. He does not prolong bed-rocking, thumb-sucking, hair-twisting; he is able to abandon such behavior as he matures.

### Level II

There is nothing very wrong here, but the differences suggest a slippage that, if unchecked, could slide on down to disease and misery. Remedial action is called for. He still laughs more than he cries and in general is a satisfactory baby, child, adolescent, adult, parent, but he has occasional moments of allergy, discontent, moodiness, sickness. His nose may run when he is on the wool rug for more than three hours. He doesn't sleep through the night until three months of age. He lollygags over breast or bottle and vomits once or twice a week when handled by a stranger. A cold develops only if someone brings it home— maybe two or three times a year—and clears rapidly with nose drops and antihistamines without accompanying ear infection.

Bouts of gas and fussiness are rare but painful and are dispelled by tea, massage, or a glycerin suppository. He is not completely satisfied on the breast and sometimes has gas if his mother eats beans, garlic, or onions. If overfed he will vomit. An occasional BM may stink.

His development matches the standard charts but he is occasionally frustrated because he crawls under a table and can't get out. He loves cuddling. He insists on sucking or rocking and needs a favorite stuffed toy at bedtime. Separation anxiety comes early—at seven or eight months—but he can be distracted out of it.

Teething may be accompanied by a fever (100° to 101°F) but aspirin is curative; no disease follows. He gets roseola but is not "sick": he just feels warm and is irritable for three days and then has a body rash and resumes smiling.

He has food preferences but can be talked into eating almost everything except liver and spinach. Rashes appear (cheeks, face, buttocks) with some new foods but disappear in a day or so. He has a hard BM only with too much rice, applesauce, or bananas.

Temper tantrums are short; he gives them up when his parents turn their backs. In a month he finds better ways to express himself: "No!" He cruises about the house touching things but seems careful and looks to his parents for approval. If they say no, he understands and does not again touch the forbidden object.

School is a little scary for a day or two but when he gets his bearings he is cooperative, a leader, and has fun. He learns easily but occasionally goes off the page and writes on his neighbor. He is sorry if he hurts someone. Only a few accidents, and never suturable cuts or concussions. He is careful with toys. Never sticks a bean up his nose. He waits to ride a bike until he is sure he can, then he does it easily. Remembers danger when warned.

Enjoys sweets but has no obvious food cravings. Accepts punishment if fair. Goes to bed with only a little reluctance.

Plays cooperatively with others. Likes to win but accepts a loss cheerfully. Doesn't care if chosen fourth when sides are picked. Defends self in a fight but will not start one. Mood swings are slight and evanescent.

Only rarely does he awaken his parents because of nocturnal fears; may wet the bed only after an exciting party or scary movie.

Adolescence is generally smooth since he has enough supportive friends and hobbies. Only twenty pimples in six years.

### Level III

The mother of the child in this category usually had a stressful pregnancy: nausea and vomiting, mild toxemia, spotty bleeding, prolonged or early or Caesarean delivery. The baby may have been premature, was slow to breathe, had to go into the incubator, perhaps also needed oxygen. Because of these factors the mother and baby are not allowed to participate in early, important mother-child interaction. She may be too weak to nurse and he may be too tired to suck, so the "helpful" nursery team puts him on cow's milk and she dries up.

He picks up weight and strength and things go well for about two to four weeks, when colic, eczema, wheeze or vomiting, gas, and diarrhea push a barely Level I baby into Level II or III. The doctor is summoned and may be able to prevent a further decline to Level IV. But these are the babies who get colic medicines, antihistamines, antibiotics, ointments, and milk changes and whose families need tranquilizers, sedatives, and aspirin.

These children are touchy, often uncuddlable—as if the world is too close. They may fight back or occasionally withdraw, suck their thumbs or rock the bed with a determination that suggests they are trying to block out a sensory overload. We want to cuddle and comfort them, but if we get too close they arch away or stiff-arm us or get so tense they will vomit—the ultimate in body language indicating rejection of our advances.

He is either terribly shy or a persistent approacher—he cannot ignore unimportant stimuli. Either environmental stimuli overwhelm him and he retreats in fear or has to attack everything that appears in his environment. Everything must go his way—no compromise, no give and take—and when sick he expects to be waited on hand and foot.

He has few friends in school, but he may be the class clown. He makes the rules for the games; he needs to win and will cheat to do it. He is a Jekyll-and-Hyde type, showing wild swings of mood. He can be very affectionate if he wants something, pouts or storms if he gets only a fair share.

He has persistent allergies. He dehydrates easily when sick.

His nights do not seem restful. He may resist going to bed. He awakens screaming with a night terror once a month, or he sleeps deeply and wets the bed. He is a grouchy bear in the morning and ruins whatever cheerful interaction his parents try to observe at breakfast. He often refuses breakfast.

You know that if he would eat properly he would feel better.

Acne is moderately severe and persistent. His hair is stringy or greasy. He doesn't seem to care. He has a bad self-image. Teachers don't like him and hope he will drop out of school; he hopes he will be expelled because he hates school anyway.

It takes a lot of social, parental, psychiatric, and medical help to keep him from juvenile delinquency. He could slip easily into a lifetime antisocial commitment.


## Level IV

Individuals unfortunate enough to qualify for this category require almost constant medical attention: daily drug therapy for epilepsy, diabetes, cystic fibrosis; gamma globulin and antibiotics to ward off infections; weekly allergy shots; antileukemia medicines; surgery for congenital anomalies, twisted bowels, kidney malfunctions, tumors, or blood clots; cortisone on a daily basis to control arthritis, colitis, nephritis, asthma. All attest to the seriousness of this level of trouble.

For many children, however, the bodies may have

arrived at this level but the emotional and intellectual level may still be up at the I and II area. Some have bodies and general physical health that qualify them for Level I or II but their psyche is at the fourth level: depression, phobias, extreme hyperactivity, belligerence, migraine.

### Level V

This category contains the bedridden, terminally ill, extremely retarded or malformed—the child about whom doctors become very depressed. We would like to help, but the conditions seem irreversible.

These levels are merely illustrative of a continuum of behavioral characteristics. Your child need not have all the characteristics of each level to force a label or cause needless concern. These profiles provide me with a general guide as to how heroic I must be with nutritional supports. Some children in Level II or III need only diet changes; others in Levels IV and V would more likely need high-potency vitamins, even injections in high doses to reverse the rapid slippage.

Parents have difficulty deciding (1) if their child is normal and as healthy as possible or (2) is off center a bit but still OK and there is nothing to worry about or (3) is really tilted and in need of some kind of help to get back to a healthy path.

We doctors see twenty to thirty patients a day and can make comparisons, but since most parents have but one or two children, how do they find out how a child is doing relative to the rest of the age group?

One doctor said the average child has four to six colds a year. But is average normal? Some children have no colds; some then must be having ten to twelve infections a year. Most of the sick infants are bottle-fed and most of the nonsick ones are breast-fed. (In a recent hospital study of one hundred infants with intestinal flu, only one was breast-fed. The La Leche League has documented many similar studies.)

The first step in making improvements in our own family's health is to accept the axiom that sickness is a clue to a malfunction in the body systems. *Few of us should get sick or have an allergy.* If we do, the immune systems and adrenal glands are cutting off. They can usually be made to work optimally with vitamins, minerals, and good nutrition.

Little problems may lead to big problems, so early intervention is prudent. A stressful or sickly pregnancy in a depressed woman may so turn her off that she will not want to or cannot nurse the baby. Every possible encouragement should be directed to nursing this baby because he is already stressed before birth.

How does one know if he or she is stressed? One person may feel a stress when another person in the same situation may feel exhilarated. I know a girl who gets canker sores. She may be feeling fine but when the blister starts to blossom, she knows someone or something has stressed her. She goes over the conversation she had with a boyfriend, what her boss said, what she ate, and the weather for the past two or three days (incubation period). "Someone did this to me!" If she could recognize the stress when it occurs, she could take extra C, B₆, calcium, and pantothenic acid and abort the canker sore.

We must change our attitudes about allergies, headaches, rashes, sleepless nights, gas, and infections. All these common (albeit minor) conditions must mean that the body is stressed and not in perfect order.

The mother of a bright, happy, busy three-year-old told me that he was the product of a comfortable sickness- and nausea-free pregnancy but was fussy and gassy in infancy when this mother consumed dairy products and then nursed him. I said "Allergy-prone children often have some history of stress that must exhaust the adrenals."

She remembered. "He was a breech baby and came

with difficulty." Could a few minutes of stress make him forever allergic? He now gets hoarse if he has four or five ounces of milk a day. Could the allergy have been precluded if extra B, C, and calcium had been given at the time of the stress on day one?

She herself is a calm, unflappable woman and took vitamin supplements and ate well during the pregnancy. She was never sick, had no nausea and a good energy level. So the difficult delivery was of only temporary concern to her mind and body, but the baby's body was stressed enough to allow the allergy to surface.

A pregnant woman with symptoms of aches and pains, nausea and vomiting, fatigue and depression must become aware that these overt symptoms require remedial action or her infant, who is sharing her body and suffering from some of the same deficiency, *may* manifest a rash, an allergy, colic, or disease susceptibility.

And what should the above-mentioned mother have done after the ideal pregnancy but stressful delivery? She took the proper path: breast-feeding. I'm convinced if she had bottle-fed the boy, he would have developed a more serious allergic condition such as eczema or asthma. The as yet unanswerable question: If the mother and the doctor had acted in a preventive way, assuming a stress had occurred, and given her and the baby some extra B complex, would the milk allergy have been avoided altogether?

I have now learned to make certain connections between the mother's pregnancy and the condition of the baby.

| If the baby has: | Mother may have had: |
|---|---|
| Cradle cap, scaly rash, cracks behind ears and in groin | Nausea and vomiting, cannot remember dreams, took the pill |

Baby may be low in $B_6$, pyridoxine

| *If the baby has:* | *Mother may have had:* |
|---|---|
| Colic, muscle cramps, insomnia, night wakefulness, milk craving, sucks, rocks, moves a lot | Backaches, muscle cramps, insomnia, menstrual cramps; loves milk or hates milk |

Baby may be low in calcium

| | |
|---|---|
| Milk and food allergy (plugged nose, gas, wheeze, rashes, etc.), ear infections, bronchitis, needs tonsil and adenoid removal | Stress and infections, allergies in family, difficult delivery; drank much milk daily in pregnancy |

Baby may be low in C, $B_6$, pantothenic acid, calcium, zinc

| | |
|---|---|
| Symptoms such as solemnity, depression, touchiness, sensitivity, allergies, wakefulness | Depression, fatigue, exhaustion after twelve hours of sleep; is anemic |

Baby may be low in $B_{12}$ and folic acid

Most parents intuitively recognize hunger, thirst, need for sleep, fatigue, potty time, depression, need for love and cuddling in their children. They usually recognize the onset of an illness. But they should know how to read the child's body well enough to treat a minor condition before it becomes major requiring the MD's services.

We learn our parents' language and the neighborhood as we grow up, but no one "teaches" us the nonverbal language of the body. If we are intuitive, we get the message.

If a patient is leaning back in the chair in my consultation room with arms folded over her chest and she has a steady inscrutable expression, I know I'm setting up negative feelings in her mind. I change my approach. I figure no matter what the treatment, she won't get well (or her child won't) unless I can change the vibrations.

If a child stops crying when I feed him, I assume he was hungry. I learn that particular cry is a hunger sound, and I can respond more accurately the next time. The autistic child who avoids eye contact and must rock or pay attention to internal sounds is telling the parents that the world or the stimuli coming into the brain are scary, and please back off.

One of our children stiff-armed us when we got too close or tried to cuddle him. If we ignored that warning sign and persisted, he threw up on us. That's a body clue that a person's space bubble has been invaded. Along with learning to read English, we must learn to read "body."

If we can take some remedial action with our children early, when the problem is usually nutritional, we should be able to reverse the trend.

The sucking, rocking, head-banging child is crying out for help. He is saying he is deficient, probably in calcium, zinc, magnesium, manganese, or B complex vitamins. But if we persist in shouting "Stop that" we are only confirming in his mind that he is a bad person. Can we look on the drug addict and the alcoholic with more empathy if we can make ourselves believe that they are trapped in their biochemistry? It is hard to call them "bad" when we realize they are the product of genetic and nutritional as well as emotional and sociological factors.

Perhaps if we learned to read children's bodies better, we could prevent them from slipping into some genetic trap. Longevity has increased in our country to the point that family disease patterns are becoming more manifest. Putting together what we see in our children with what we know runs in the family, we can get some nutritional guidelines for any child's life that should lead to health and longevity.

If grandparents have diabetes and obesity and the child is heavy and loves sweets, an effort should be made to keep quick carbohydrates out of the house and get him to think brewer's yeast is as important as pure air.

If allergies are rampant in the family, think several times before bringing a cat home as a pet.

If everyone is sensitive, goosey, and ticklish, it would be best to live in a big house out in the country and drink raw milk.

Following is a list of symptoms a child might display and what those symptoms could mean. Use your common sense and also ask your child questions. Check with your doctor. Some of these require expert medical attention; some need only domestic detective work.

| *Ask:* | *What it may mean:* |
| --- | --- |
| Do you hurt? | |
| Headaches | Low blood sugar due to allergy or sugar ingestion |
| Muscle aches<br>Growing pains<br>Menstrual cramps | Low calcium or magnesium |
| Stomachaches. Does it come and go? | Food allergy or virus intestinal flu |
| Joint pains | Arthritis: injury, allergy, inflammation |
| Burning, itching about anus | Pinworms, food allergy, constipation |
| Burning, stinging on urination<br>Frequency of urination | Infection, allergy to food or drink |
| Itchy, burning skin | Allergy to food, soap, or clothes |
| Cold when others OK | Low thyroid function, hypoglycemia |
| Scared, depressed, tired, can't concentrate | Hypoglycemia, anemia, food allergy, anxiety, need vitamin B$_3$ (500 to 2000 mg) |
| Think better in the A.M., spacy after school lunch | Hypoglycemia, food allergy, tough teacher |
| Favorite food? | |
| Sweets | Hypoglycemia |
| Coffee, chocolate, cola (caffeine) | Hypoglycemia |
| Milk | Low calcium |

| *Ask:* | *What it may mean:* |
|---|---|
| Salt | Low in vitamins and minerals generally, zinc specifically |
| Trouble falling asleep | Low calcium, magnesium, zinc, manganese |
| Ticklish, sensitive, unable to disregard unimportant things | Low calcium, genetic trait, birth injury, low in B complex, especially $B_6$ |
| If more restless after a loading dose of B vitamins | Low calcium |
| Trouble getting up in A.M. | Usually need protein at bedtime. Hypoglycemia, anemia, low thyroid |

| *If you see:* | *It may mean:* |
|---|---|
| Pallor | Anemia, allergy, hypoglycemia, low thyroid, sick, about to vomit |
| Dark circles under eyes | Food allergy |
| Eczema | Food allergy, low vitamin A and zinc, exhausted adrenal glands |
| Hives, itchy rashes | Allergen ingested plus stress, exhausted adrenals, scabies |
| Dermatographia, scaly scalp, dandruff, cracks behind ears, groin rash | Seborrhea (may need $B_6$); food allergy (often milk); low calcium, pantothenic acid |
| Acne | Low zinc, low vitamin A, food allergy, high iodine intake (kelp, seafood) |
| Rocking, foot-swinging, nail-biting, thumb-sucking, bed-rocking, hair-twisting, hand-shaking. Any rhythmical, repetitive tension-relieving activity | Low calcium, magnesium, low vitamin D, low manganese, low zinc; insecure, afraid, bored, sensitive |
| Eye blinking, squinting, red white matter, crusting, itching | Low vitamin A, $B_2$, C; food allergy; need eye exam |

| *If you see:* | *It may mean:* |
|---|---|
| Big pupils, trembling, frightened, withdrawn, night terrors | Excess adrenalin from low blood sugar or food allergy; stress |
| Falling hair; nails cracked, split; soft, ridged white spots | Low-protein diet, stress, low $B_6$; low zinc, calcium, vitamin A |
| Rubs, picks nose | Allergy, usually inhalation |
| Watery mucus from nose | Allergy, usually inhalation |
| Green or yellow exudate from nose | Secondary infection |
| Wandering about at night, restless sleep, tearing up bed, night terrors, sleep walking | Excess adrenalin from low blood sugar or food allergy; stress; low calcium, low magnesium, low zinc, manganese |
| Small bladder capacity, bed wetting | Hypoglycemia, food allergy, low magnesium |

| *If you hear:* | *It may mean:* |
|---|---|
| Snorting, sniffling, zonking, throat-clearing | Milk allergy, food allergy, inhalation allergy, big adenoids |
| Sneezing | Inhalation allergy |
| Gas | Food allergy, low digestive enzymes, low stomach acid, unfriendly bacteria |
| Head-hanging, bed-rocking, night screaming, talking, restlessness | Hypoglycemia, food allergy, low calcium, low magnesium, low vitamin D |
| Sighing | Low calcium, magnesium, vitamin D; stress |
| Odd noises when urine hits toilet-bowl water | Infection, allergy, injury, anomaly |

| *If you feel:* | *It may mean:* |
|---|---|
| Tight muscle, spastic, tender to touch | Low calcium, low magnesium, injury, acidosis, fatigue, low potassium, neurological problem, disease inside (appendicitis, cellulitis) |

| *If you feel:* | *It many mean:* |
|---|---|
| Pulse rapid | Exercise, emotion, food allergy, falling blood sugar, bleeding, fever |
| Pulse slow | Good health, low thyroid, heart anomalies |
| Rough skin (nutmeg-grater feel to skin on back of arms and thighs) | Hyperkeratosis or low vitamin A |
| Dry skin | Low in vitamins A, E, and fatty acids |
| Cold, dry hands and feet | Low thyroid, low iodine |
| Cold, moist palms | Anxiety, hypoglycemia, food allergy |
| Swollen glands: | |
| Back of neck | Sinus, postnasal drip, milk allergy, dandruff, scalp infection |
| Under corner of jawbone | Throat or tonsil infection |
| Armpit, groin | Skin infection or irritation nearby |

| *If you smell:* | *It may mean:* |
|---|---|
| Bad breath | Infection in nose, mouth, throat, lungs; food fermenting in intestines and smelly gases carried to lungs; digestive enzymes not working |
| Much gas being passed | Much air swallowing |
| Passing smelly gas | Food fermenting; food allergy |
| Passing rotten-egg smell | Salmonella, low vitamin C |
| Ears: smell of old cheese or dirty socks | Fungus; low zinc, vitamin A and C |
| Bad body odor despite bathing | Low zinc, low vitamin A |
| Putrid odor from any opening | Foreign object causing infection (especially in the nose) |
| Unusual odor in urine | Food allergy; rare metabolic disease (e.g., PKU); urine infection |

# The Quality 2 Pregnancy

Many women have stressful pregnancies, difficult deliveries, and perfect children. Many women have comfortable pregnancies, easy deliveries, but are burdened with a colicky, touchy and allergic child. Usually, however, a stressless well-nourished pregnancy that culminates in an easy delivery nets a content, easy-to-rear, healthy child.

With the help of an experienced midwife or obstetrician "reading the pregnancy" should allow the participants to reorganize the internal and external environments of mother and baby. Stress, drugs, and poor nutrition are common factors that may lead to sickness, allergies, and physical and mental defects that may plague a child for the rest of his life.

| Symptom or sign | Could lead to: | Try this to relieve: |
|---|---|---|
| Nausea and vomiting in early pregnancy | Exhaustion, malnutrition, seborrhea, colic, learning disabilities | $B_6$, nibbling on nuts, cheese, protein |

| Symptom or sign | Could lead to: | Try this to relieve: |
| --- | --- | --- |
| Muscle cramps, backache | Painful delivery | Calcium, magnesium, manganese, potassium |
| Stretch marks | Stretch marks | Vitamin E, A, zinc |
| Gas | Discomfort | Change diet, acidophilus |
| Fatigue | Exhaustion, depression, inability to nurse | B complex, $B_{12}$, folic acid |
| Edema, swollen ankles | High blood pressure, toxemia | Protein diet, $B_6$, salt (fluid needed for nursing) |
| Headaches | Fatigue and depression | Nibbling on protein and vegetables, no sugar |
| Gaining too much | Fatigue (if due to unrefined carbohydrates) | Nibbling on protein and vegetables, 25 to 30 lbs. best for 9 months |
| Gaining too little | Undernourished baby | Add vitamins B, C, calcium and minerals. May benefit from vitamin shots. |
| Food cravings Smoking Alcohol ingestion Drugs | Malnutrition | B complex (50 to 100 mg of each of Bs), calcium 2000 mg, magnesium 800 to 1000 mg, raw vegetables, seeds, nuts, brewer's yeast, kelp |
| Excessive intra-uterine activity | Allergic or hyperactive child | Stop milk and foods eaten daily. Use 4-day rotation diet. Add calcium |
| Sinusitis, increase in allergies, | Allergic child | Plan to nurse, use calcium, extra C, |

| Symptom or sign | Could lead to: | Try this to relieve: |
|---|---|---|
| rashes, wheezes | | B, pantothenic acid, eliminate milk |

*Nausea and vomiting* during the pregnancy does not have to mean a psychological rejection of the child. It is usually caused by a low B₆ (pyridoxine) level in the body. The liver needs this vitamin to metabolize the excess female hormones. (Since $B_6$ is necessary for memory, inability to remember dreams, for example, would be one confirmatory clue that $B_6$ is deficient.) Low blood sugar in the morning would tend to trigger the nausea. A pregnant woman should eat some protein substance right at bedtime and have some left to eat first thing in the morning. Nausea and vomiting could be the initial event leading to a miserable, fatiguing pregnancy. The resulting baby may be allergic, have seborrhea (cradle cap), and colic because of a milk allergy. Pregnancy exhaustion might preclude satisfactory nursing.

*Treatment:* Protein snacks, especially those high in the B complex vitamins, should be consumed every two to three hours. Pregnancy is no time for a woman to go on a weight-loss diet. Weight gain is best at twenty-five to thirty-five pounds or more for the nine months. The baby is nourished with the vitamins, minerals, amino acids, oxygen, and water flowing through its mother's bloodstream, not by what is stored. $B_6$ at the 50-to-100-mg-per-day dose or intramuscular shots of $B_6$ should control nausea.

*Threatened miscarriage* with cramps and bleeding could be a mechanical problem (relaxed opening of the uterus, placenta attached low in uterus) but some are related to low levels of vitamin E and possibly vitamin C.

If a threatened miscarriage becomes a premature birth, a whole set of new stresses and allergies and other risks may surface. The uterus is the best incubator.

*Treatment:* Bed rest makes sense. The doctor's advice should be followed, but a supernourishing diet plus extra vitamin E (400 to 800 units) and vitamin C (500 to 2000 mg) and foods containing these vitamins should be taken. Calcium and magnesium should have a calming effect on the uterine muscles.

*Stress* to the mother (or what she perceives as a stress) or to the baby at birth would contribute to development of allergies, infection, and even hyperactivity. A long labor, difficult delivery, or Caesarean section could exhaust the mother and possibly interfere with her ability to hold, nurse, and bond with her baby after delivery.

*Treatment:* Stress exhausts the adrenal glands, so some effort should be made to both treat and think preventively. The doctor can give the mother 5 to 10 grams of vitamin C intravenously at the end of any anesthesia used. He can order vitamin B complex injections to be given daily to help restore the mother's mind and body. If an IV is needed, it should contain amino acids instead of dextrose; the body needs restorative protein, not just energy.

If the mother can be encouraged to nurse despite her fatigue, the baby may avoid an allergic life. If it is not possible, goat's milk (raw certified is best) might be the best second choice.

If the baby shows any symptom of developing colic, restlessness, insomnia, or uncuddlability, the assumption can be made that the baby's adrenal glands suffered the stress along with the mother and should be helped with the B complex also.

*Postpartum depression* is frequently treated psychiatrically but is now believed to be a combination of hormone withdrawal, low blood sugar, and possibly some emotional forces.

*Treatment:* It is amazing how a shot of $B_{12}$ can often reverse the process overnight. (I use 0.4 cc of Folbesyn® by Lederle Company, which has the B complex and folic acid, plus 0.4 cc of $B_{12}$ that comes 1000 mcg per cc. It is given intramuscularly about every other day for two weeks and then a decision is made as to the frequency of injections after that.) The baby's interest should be considered also. If the B vitamins help the mother, the baby is probably suffering from the same deficiencies. I don't know if there is a way of predicting which woman is going to have the problem: perhaps the one who notices premenstrual tension or has had some depressive episode for no good reason. Taking extra B vitamins (capsule, injections, brewer's yeast, foods containing B vitamins) before and after delivery should reduce the likelihood of postpartum depression. Of course, a supportive family and medical back-up system would help. Ask your doctor.

### Questions and Answers

**Q. I am pregnant with lots of nausea and vomiting and insomnia. I don't eat junk before bedtime. What can I do?**

**A.** Pregnant women with those symptoms are frequently low in vitamin $B_6$. The insomnia may be due to low calcium. Your baby is subject to the same deficiencies and could develop cradle cap, colic, and insomnia also. Try to nibble on protein every two to three hours. If a pregnant woman does not eat supper, she will have acetone in her urine in the morning—a sign that fat is being used for energy.

**Q. Should I drink four or more glasses of milk a day? I hate it.**

**A.** Milk supplies calcium and vitamins and is a good

protein source, but there are other ways to get all these things into the body. We all need about 1000 mg of calcium a day, and about double that for a pregnant woman. Use cheese, sesame seeds, lots of greens, and herb teas with calcium plus oystershell calcium plus magnesium and vitamin D.

**Q. My obstetrician wants me to gain no more than twenty to twenty-five pounds for the whole nine months. I'm six months along and have already gained that. I can't face him.**

A. He's not keeping up on research in the last twenty years. Women do better if they gain a minimum of fifteen to twenty pounds by five months and then about two pounds a month after that. The woman's blood volume increases by 50 percent, and if she does not get enough protein, water, and salt to fill that space, she may get toxemia, a deficiency disease.

Tell him you are sorry but you want your baby well nourished. And don't let him prescribe a water pill.

**Q. I'm allergic to dairy products, wheat, and eggs. If I stay away from them during the pregnancy, will my baby not develop an allergy to them?**

A. Possibly. Allergies seem to be less noticeable when people follow the four-day rotation diet. That is, don't eat any food more frequently than once every four or five days. However, knowing about the family allergies, you would be wise to restrict the consumption of these foods and increase your intake of the foods and nutrients that make the adrenals function properly (vitamin C, B$_6$, pantothenic acid, calcium, vitamin A, and zinc). Lentils and beans are a good source of protein.

A woman told me that her baby was diagnosed as being allergic to cow's milk in the second day of life and was given soy milk for six to eight months. I asked about a stress that might have exhausted the adrenal glands of both mother and child. She denied any problem. But she loved milk and drank two quarts a day.

It would have been wise, in retrospect, if she had consumed dairy products only every fourth day and taken the extra D, C, and B vitamins and calcium. Nursing the baby is the best method of avoiding the problem.

**Q. I worry about the large doses of vitamins and minerals you recommend in your book, Feed Your Kids Right. I'm afraid that they could damage the baby. How can I be sure?**

**A.** They are safe. Be sure to take at least the recommended daily allowance that the government suggests as a minimum. Then take another look at your body. The symptoms and signs are clues that stress or poor nutrition is present. Your body may have special needs due to the quality of your mother's pregnancy with you.

If you drink a quart of milk a day and still have muscle cramps, you are probably not getting enough calcium (or salt) or you are allergic to milk, and because of that rejection you cannot absorb the calcium from milk. Swallowing is not the same as absorbing. Does it seem unsafe to you to get your calcium from tablets, dolomitic limestone (check to see that dolomite compound is free of any metal contaminants; if you have any doubts, use another type of calcium supplement), bone meal, or oyster shells rather than the cow? Your ancestors chewed on bones. Are you really that much different? The purpose of eating is to supply the body with the vitamins and minerals it needs to function properly.

Our topsoil is becoming deficient. Even if we eat well, it is not a guarantee that we will get the minimum amounts of minerals our bodies must have to function properly.

# The Delivery 3
## and the Newborn

If the pregnancy has been comfortable, free from stress and allergies, and the mother has not been sick, has eaten well, gained twenty-five to thirty pounds or more, and had only an occasional drink of wine and an aspirin or two, the baby should be full-term, pink, alert, eager to nurse, and fun to cuddle. If the family background is full of diabetes, obesity, allergies, and susceptibility to infections, then special attention should be made during the pregnancy to avoid sugar, white-flour products, and junk in general and to take extra B complex vitamins, vitamin C, and an all-purpose mineral supplement.

If allergies are a prominent familial feature, the prudent pregnant woman should attempt the four-day rotation diet and plan to nurse her baby for at least a year. Thinking ahead might preclude an allergy. Some pregnant women will drink milk every Monday and Friday and take calcium and magnesium on the off days. This will assure her and the baby of the necessary amounts of the bone and teeth minerals but will cut down on the allergic load—for both of them. It would be a good rule to follow also when nursing. An allergy to the cow's milk that the mother is drinking is the most common cause of colic in the breast-fed baby.

If the pregnancy was satisfactory but the delivery was a stress, maybe the mother should take extra B complex and vitamin C for a few days: a B complex with 50 to 100 mg of each of the Bs and 1000 to 10,000 mg of vitamin C per day (depending on the looseness of the bowels). If she gets the postpartum blues, a couple of $B_{12}$ shots may clear it up in two to three days.

If possible, the birth process should be stressless. It is obviously hard work, but if the parents have been working through and with a natural childbirth education group, or with the Lamaze and the La Leche League support teams, then the whole effort can be like training for and winning at the Olympics, and for a better prize. These groups are in every major city and anxious to smooth the way.

But how does any first-time pregnant woman know what is best for her and her baby? Is she going to the "right" doctor or midwife? An accoucheur should be flexible enough to be able to vary his "standard" method of delivery to accommodate his "unique" patient. What works for some may not work for others. But the clues are there.

A close-to-term pregnant woman should take 1000 to 5000 mg of vitamin C, 100 mg of each of the Bs, and 1000 to 2000 mg of calcium daily just in case some unexpected stress arises during delivery. When in doubt about what is happening to the mother before, during or after the delivery, assume her body needs supportive nutrients.

| Symptom or sign | Could lead to: | May be alleviated by: |
|---|---|---|
| Long, hard labor | Exhaustion and depression in mother and allergy in baby, sick baby, problems nursing | Vitamin C, B complex, calcium |
| Fever or infection | (similar problems to above) | Vitamin C, fluids, antibiotics, rest |
| Postpartum depression | Hospitalization, inability to nurse, poor attachment process with baby | B$_{12}$ injection, folic acid, no-sugar diet |
| Heavy flow | Anemia | Vitamin A, C, bioflavenoids, nursing |
| Inadequate milk supply | Discouragement, non-nursing, poor weight gain | Vitamin B (50–100 mg of each), 4–5 T. brewer's yeast per day, extra fluid, rest, encouragement |
| Sneezing (mother or baby) | Usually an inhalant allergy | Air purifier, no animals, no wool or down in the room |
| Twitches, jerks, convulsions (in baby) | Serious illness (see the doctor; get blood tests) | Calcium, magnesium, manganese, B$_6$ |

Developing the good self-image begins as soon as the baby is born, and it helps if the delivery has been quiet and as comfortable as possible. Ideally the mother can cuddle the baby against her chest, the baby is alert enough to suck, and the father is beaming and stroking. One father told me he was able to hold his newly born daughter while his wife was being "pulled together."

This tiny newborn was searching with eyes and ears as if lost on a foggy night looking and listening for signs of home. Her dad began to talk. "Your mother's busy now, but she will be with you soon. She's a nice lady and you'll like her. I'm your dad, and we'll get to know each other very well. We have your room and bed all fixed. It's yellow because we didn't know. . . ." Twenty minutes.

The interesting but hardly surprising result was that for the next eight months when her father came home and shouted "I'm home!" this girl would stop whatever she was doing, look and listen. That man is an important part of her life.

These blobs of protoplasm are obviously more than a loud noise at one end and no responsibility at the other. They are taking notes; they file things away in their computer storage cells. If, however, they are uncomfortable, sensitive, goosey, they may get a distorted perception that the world is a menace.

It is important that we make these infants as comfortable as possible. We cannot perceive their perceptions, but they are giving us clues so we can help them.

### Questions and Answers

**Q. My doctor wants to deliver me in the hospital, but I would like a home delivery. Can I get my way?**

**A.** Your doctor is telling you he is trained for and comfortable with hospital-based deliveries. You are probably stuck with what your community offers. Many hospitals now have homelike rooms attached to the hospital so if something goes awry, the woman can be wheeled through to the "science" place. You should at least insist on having your mate-coach with you during the labor and delivery. It makes sense.

There are risks to home deliveries; when an emergency arises, quick action may be required to save the mother and the baby.

Q. Why is the rate of Caesarean sections going up? I'd just as soon not have one. Do I have a choice?

A. It is true; the rate is getting higher and ranges from 10 to 40 percent. It may be related to the doctors' training, but it may be that they want to interrupt a long and stressful labor. It is also possible that modern women are less likely to have an adequate pelvis. This could be from generations of poor diet according to Weston Price in *Nutrition and Physical Degeneration.*

Q. My last labor was very painful. Can I take something that is not a drug or narcotic?

A. It doesn't always work, but about 2000 mg of calcium in some form might be helpful. Muscles low in calcium are more responsive to irritation and tend to cramp more. Try dolomite (not absorbed too well) or some other calcium-magnesium combination, or calcium lactate just when labor sets in. Vitamin C at about the 1000-mg level every hour helps the body handle stress; C acts on the brain to take the sharp edge off the pain.

Q. I'm scheduled for a home delivery as I have babies easily and have a competent accoucheur. My three-and-a-half-year-old boy knows there is a baby inside. Should I let him watch?

A. Most children who are in attendance are fascinated and seem to take it all very objectively but get bored occasionally. Give him the option. "You're welcome, but if you want to watch TV, we'll call you when the baby is here." If you become very sick or distressed, he probably should be escorted elsewhere.

### The Newborn

A mother should try to nurse her baby, even if only for a short period of time. In order for her to be ready for this, her pregnancy should be as stressless and well-nourished as possible. No drugs, especially the water pills, should be used.

If a woman delivers in a hospital, she should insist that no feedings—except a swallow of water—be given to her baby in the nursery. She should be as tough and demanding as she must to keep her baby close to her. It would be wise if she and the baby can get back home quickly so the baby can be nursed on demand.

One of the chief reasons for a home delivery or rooming-in plan is to allow the mother and baby to be close as early as possible after the delivery. This helps to promote the nursing and, of course, is important in establishing the bonding more effectively. If the baby can be applied to the breast very soon after delivery, the baby will receive the colostrum, which is full of immunity-building material. The mother's uterus returns to normal size more rapidly if she nurses. Human babies are not allergic to human milk.

Most doctors used to discourage nursing because they did not realize the tremendous advantages of breast over bottle. They worried that the breast milk would be insufficient; at least they could count the number of ounces consumed from the bottle.

We now know breast milk is the best possible milk for the baby. Grandparents can help during the pregnancy with subtle hints: "You will nurse your baby, won't you, dear?" The La Leche League should be contacted well before the due date so techniques can be learned and motivation developed. If the doctor tends to discourage nursing, the mother should smile politely but ignore him. Nursing is especially important for a baby who comes from allergic parents. It is also necessary to remember that foods the mother eats can get into her milk and cause gas, bloat, rashes, and colic in her baby. The simplest way to demonstrate this is for the nursing mother to eat a tuna sandwich with chopped green onions. It takes about thirty to sixty minutes for the ingested irritant to get into the mother's milk and about a day to go from the baby's stomach until it is finally passed rectally.

Most babies lose some weight in the first few days. This is some extra fluid and has little significance. The birth weight should be regained by the tenth to fourteenth day. Once they start to gain they usually pick up about 4 ounces a week or a minimum of a pound per month. Most nursing mothers who feel that their breast milk is inadequate can sometimes increase the amount by the ingestion of the stress formula of C, B complex, and calcium as mentioned above.

Even adopted babies can be nursed. It takes dedication and determination, but with the help of the La Leche League and the Lactaid device some milk usually shows up in a week or so. A message from the nipples travels up to the brain saying "There's a baby out there." The brain cannot understand why the uterus didn't say anything but goes ahead with the lactogenic hormone anyway. Babies put up for adoption are more likely to have suffered prenatal stress and seem to have a higher incidence of allergies.

If the mother would recall the events of her pregnancy, then she should be able to deduce the reason for the baby's symptoms or signs.

| Symptom or sign | Suggests or Could lead to: | May be alleviated by: |
|---|---|---|
| Pimply rash on face | Food allergy to something the mother ate before birth | Time, food avoidance |
| Seborrhea, oily yellow scales, cracks under ears, groin; rash | Usually means mother had nausea and vomiting. Child can be colicky or allergic | $B_6$ in B complex orally, vitamin E rubbed into scales may help |
| Colic—crying that is not | Allergy to cow's milk or, if nurs- | Changing milk (don't stop nurs- |

| Symptom or sign | Suggests or Could lead to: | May be alleviated by: |
|---|---|---|
| caused by hunger | ing, cow's milk the mother drank, discouragement | ing), adding calcium, zinc, manganese, $B_6$, herbal teas, potassium; try a suppository for tight anal ring |
| Watery nose, phlegm in throat, cough | Allergy to cow's milk or, if nursing, something the mother ate | Changing milk (don't stop nursing); vitamin C and pantothenic acid |

### Questions and Answers

Q. I'm nursing my baby, who is two weeks old. I worry that she is not getting enough. She nurses for twenty minutes every two hours, then drops off into deep sleep. She does sleep six hours at night.

A. Don't change a thing! That's ideal. If she can get her twenty-four-hour requirements swallowed in eighteen hours, you are way ahead. She will soon sleep eight hours, then ten, then twelve hours when she stops growing so fast.

Q. My boy is three weeks old and his gas is getting worse. We use Enfamil with iron.

A. Everyone who eats has gas; much of it is swallowed air. Incomplete digestion can lead to fermentation. If the gas causes pain, you might try plain Enfamil. Iron can be an irritant and may not be effective in preventing anemia until he is five to seven months old. If that's no good, try soybean milk. Don't give up.

Q. My baby is breast-fed and gaining well but is constipated. She has a bowel movement every five to seven days. Should I use a suppository daily?

A. Constipation is determined by the consistency

and not the frequency. Breast-fed babies absorb the milk so well there is less to pass but what does come, usually every three to seven days, is yellow and like thick soup. It has a not unpleasant yeasty smell. You're doing great.

**Q. Our baby boy is but two weeks old and seems to require extra sucking beyond what he gets from the bottle. Is a pacifier OK?**

**A.** Breast-fed babies have to work harder to get their milk, which may be a reason for the more even teeth and better dental arch but may explain why bottle-fed babies are more likely to need the pacifier and may end up as "tongue thrusters." The pacifier (Nuk® is better) will push the teeth around less than thumb or fingers and may be easier to stop at age five or six. Some of those who love to suck are probably very sensitive people and are trying to "block" the uncomfortable sensory messages from the world and their busy intestines. It is *not* a sign of insecurity or anxiety. Some need calcium.

# Birth 4 to Six Months

By the time babies are four to six weeks of age they usually sleep through the night. They have been growing at a fantastic rate, and those who are destined to be large adults and those with colic will still be up at night. Most will gain about two pounds a month in the first half year.

A large number of breast-fed babies seem to have trouble sleeping through the night. One explanation might be that the milk is so completely absorbed and utilized it has no long-term "holding" power and the baby is hungry every two to three hours. Some will find early feeding of solids in the evening is helpful.

If the doctor (or a relative) suggests the introduction of solid foods for no specific reason, try to disregard the advice as it will serve no useful purpose and may initiate food allergies.

If breast-feeding is out of the question, raw goat's milk may be the best substitute for the human type—if you know the goat is healthy. Goat's milk is deficient in folic acid, so that must be supplemented. After that might come Enfamil®, Similac®, SMA®, and other prepared cow's milks. (Because of processing they are less allergenic than raw cow's milk.) To gain weight and do well babies usually consume two ounces for every pound of body weight per twenty-four hours. That's easy to figure out if a bottle is used, but a breast-fed baby may have to be weighed weekly. If a breast-fed baby is urinating at least three times a day and can go without nursing for at least one four- to six-hour period in twenty-four hours, he or she is probably getting enough.

If the baby develops any of the following conditions, some remedial action is called for.

*Colic and night wakefulness;* wants small feedings every two hours; mother had muscle cramps. There may be a deficiency of calcium.

*Colic and sneezing,* watery nose, cough and wheeze, eczema, and explosive diarrhea; family has allergies. Mother had stress in pregnancy or childbirth. Probably exhausted adrenal glands, which leads to allergies. *Treatment:* Change whatever milk is being used (don't stop nursing but stop the cow's milk, cheese and the like, the mother is eating, change to soy, goat, meat base if baby is bottle-fed); help adrenals with vitamin C, $B_6$, pantothenic acid, vitamin A, calcium, and zinc. Herb teas that have calcium and pantothenic acid should help (comfrey, dandelion, parsley, alfalfa).

A baby who does not like to cuddle or stiff-arms loving parents, dislikes closeness, needs to rock or suck, and fights sleep may be allergic to something but is more likely low in a mineral (calcium, magnesium, zinc, or manganese). If the B vitamins seem to stimulate the baby, it suggests a histamine release; these infants (and children or adults) usually need calcium.

A colicky, fussy, gassy, squirming baby with a red

bottom (where urine hits) is usually allergic to milk, orange juice, or color additives in the vitamins. If the redness is confined to the area between the buttocks around the anal opening, it is usually due to peaches, eggs, wheat or something solid recently added to the diet. It may be a reaction to food or milk, but not a soap or diaper rash. Eat it today, wear it tomorrow. A yeast infection may look like a food allergy.

*Treatment:* Most doctors will supply a sample of a cortisone-containing cream, which is anti-inflammatory and antiallergic. If this helps, assume that the baby's adrenals have been stressed and add vitamin C, $B_6$, pantothenic acid, calcium, vitamin A, and zinc while experimenting with the diet. Adding acidophilus to the diet may alter the intestinal bacteria enough to promote digestion and absorption so the foods will not leak out and irritate the skin.

Vitamins are present in fresh human and animal milk, and the commercial varieties have had some added. These may be adequate unless a "reading" of the body indicates that a slippage from the ideal has occurred. It is probably better to use cod-liver oil as the infant's source of vitamin A (5000 to 10,000 units per day) and D (500 to 1000 units per day) than the vitamins in a base with sugar, color, and flavorings.

The most convenient form of vitamin C for a baby is sodium ascorbate (the sodium salt of ascorbic acid) powder, since it is not as sour as the acids. A teaspoon has 4000 to 5000 mg, so just a pinch in some water would be adequate for the normal baby (100 mg per day). Using C alone would make it easy on stress days, when parents would want to increase the amount of C without increasing the other vitamins unnecessarily; for the immunizations it would be prudent to give the baby 500 to 1000 mg of vitamin C the day before, the day of, and the day following the shots.

Vitamin C could be similarly increased when the weather changes, when there has been exposure to infections, or when the baby appears to be coming down with a virus or an allergy. Some parents experiment with the dose until the baby shows some increased sloppiness in bowel movements (which may be hard to detect in a breast-fed baby). Then they cut back and give this saturation dose daily. When stress strikes, the daily dose would be given hourly until a day or so after the stress of infection has disappeared. It is best to taper off.

I used to think this dosage was excessive. But now, after many years of treating children with antibiotics and other drugs, I believe the strong vitamin C approach is infinitely safer, easier, and cheaper than the standard medical approach. The latter may be necessary, however, and can certainly be used simultaneously. Follow your doctor's recommendations.

The B complex vitamins would be necessary if highly processed milk is being given; a breast-fed baby has no extra need unless the mother is under great stress or is on a deficient diet, or the baby shows some allergy or is sick.

Extra calcium seems superfluous unless the baby has excessive rhythmical activities, insomnia that cannot be controlled with a diet change, or seems overly responsive to lights and sounds. Magnesium deficiencies are often related. A safe dose to try on a three- to six-week-old baby is about 100 to 200 mg of calcium plus 50 to 100 mg of magnesium per day at bedtime for a week.

A breast-fed baby gets all the necessary vitamins and minerals from a well-nourished mother. Cod-liver oil drops probably should be given to babies in the winter in smoggy cities in the North.

### Questions and Answers

**Q. Why would a breast-fed baby scream constantly, wanting to nurse every hour and a half? The doctor said to wait three to four hours.**

A. The doctor doesn't remember how hungry he was at that age. If a baby continued to grow at the rate he does in the first two to three weeks, by the time he was ten years old he would be twenty feet tall. Assume he is hungry and feed him. The stomach empties in one and a half to two hours. If he is unhappy all the time, it could be caused by something in *your* diet.

Q. How long would it take for a food the nursing mother eats to get into the baby and cause an upset?

A. Usually just half an hour to two hours is all. It takes about twenty-four hours to go through the mother's (and the baby's) intestines, so both may be unhappy all that time. Garlic, onions, beans, cabbage, and the like are possible causes—but remember the motto of the allergists: "Anything can do anything."

Q. Why does my baby always wake up crying?

A. Many people when very hungry (blood sugar dropping rapidly) release adrenalin from the adrenals. The adrenalin often makes them feel frightened: "An all-gone feeling." "Spacey." "A sensation of impending doom." Allergenic foods (possibly milk) may release histamine, which stimulates the nervous system.

Q. My baby is four months old and sleeps through the night, thank God. But he screams most of the day. Help!

A. If he eats every hour and gets his twenty-four-hour quota ingested in twelve hours and then sleeps all night, it's just hunger. But it may be the chemical flavoring, coloring, or sugar in the vitamins you give him in the morning that makes him uncomfortable all day. Check the labels on the vitamins and switch to a brand that doesn't have these additives, if necessary. Or, if you are nursing him, it may be something you eat for breakfast that gets into your milk and cramps him until bedtime.

Q. Does colic affect the personality makeup later on?

**A.** Colic is a clue that the child is sensitive and may grow to be a hyperactive child and a restless adult. But many colicky babies become sweet, gentle, easy-to-live-with adults. The problem is more how parents can handle their own reactions to the constant screaming. In spite of the stresses evoked by the noise and lack of sleep, parents have to communicate to the child that he is loved and accepted.

**Q. Do you think colic is a real disease? If so, what is the treatment?**

**A.** About twenty things could explain the painful cramps. It could be a normal amount of gas going sideways in a baby who is sensitive and notices everything. The mother nursing a colicky baby should eat—for only a day or two—the usual safe foods: rice, applesauce, bananas, lamb, and yellow vegetables. If that doesn't help, 100 to 300 mg of calcium a day may calm the poor thing. A variety of herbal teas have been found effective, probably because they contain calcium, potassium, pantothenic acid, and some B vitamins—all the nutrients that help support the adrenals and help the brain be less sensitive to incoming stimuli.

If a baby on formula is calmed in two days on soy or goat's milk, an allergy is assumed to be present, and an effort should be made to minimize exposure to common allergens (no animals, wool, feathers; delay solid food introduction).

Colic associated with infrequent urination could be a result of urinary-tract obstruction. A tight anal ring may explain discomfort at bowel-movement time.

**Q. Why would a totally breast-fed baby spit up many times a day and not sleep through the night?**

**A.** Doctors used to call these babies hypertonic and stone them with sedatives. Some of them became hyperactive—restless, never-satisfied insomniacs. I would assume something in your diet every day (milk, vitamins, eggs, wheat, corn) is getting through and irritating the baby's stomach. Calcium may be needed; try more yourself (1 to 2 grams per day and 100 to 400 mg for the baby; a mixture of oystershell calcium, zinc, magnesium, and manganese with vitamin D should be ideal). Calcium is usually given at bedtime for its calming effect. Health stores now carry a liquid calcium that can be dripped down the throat.

## Colic (crying that is not due to hunger)

*Breast-fed*

Not enough milk; allergic to mother's diet (milk, vitamins, onions, beans, etc.); bad position; colic and seborrhea (cradle cap, scaly rash); mother had nausea and vomiting—may be a $B_6$ deficiency

*Bottle-fed*

Holes in nipple too small or too large; sensitive to being held (try propping); tight anal sphincter (try suppository); sensitive to milk protein or the sugar (try raw goat's or soybean milk)

# Six Months 5
## to One Year

Most parents can begin to breathe easily once their child is about six or seven months of age, has shown no major allergies, has not been sick, appears to be developing normally, is sleeping through the night and laughs more than cries. A great kid.

Many women will decide to stop nursing ("Your breasts will be down to your kneecaps!"). Within a month of the switchover to cow's milk (often homogenized and pasteurized) the baby may develop a cold and subsequent bronchial or ear infections, become constipated (cow's milk is the most common cause), or blossom out with an ugly rash or eczema (milk is the prime allergen).

It is so clear to me that this sequence represents an allergic response to cow's milk that I have trouble understanding many pediatricians' reluctance to act on this obvious body clue. The cow's milk must be stopped immediately and goat or soy milk substituted, the stress of separation minimized, and sugar in the diet eliminated.

The nutrients for the obviously exhausted adrenals should be increased.

I try to encourage women who wish to discontinue nursing for whatever reason to be ever so gradual in the substitution. Maybe an ounce a day of cow's milk can be added; then observe any reaction. If there is none, the cow's milk can be increased and the nursing discouraged. (I am writing this as if the baby had no part in the decision-making process. Some will set up so many objections to the loss of oral pleasure, either verbally or physically, that many mothers postpone the changeover.) If nursing stops totally and the baby falls apart with infections and allergies, the best milk source is lost. Do it gradually. If a problem develops, one can usually return to the safety of the best milk for humans.

Every age has some associated stress. The six- to twelve-month-old is rapidly learning about gravity, people, temperature, texture. He is cutting teeth. He suddenly realizes that he is not attached to his mother and she disappears occasionally. Strangers may seem too close and threatening. Not everyone pays attention when he pat-a-cakes. He may not get his diapers changed the minute they are soiled. He may not be fed at the first hunger pain. Frustrations are daily occurrences. All these stresses may lead to sickness for an infant with poor ability to cope. Don't push the child. It may look like an easy age to us, but to the six- to twelve-month-old, life is pretty scary, albeit exciting. Making too many food changes may be the trigger that initiates sickness.

No solids should be introduced until well after six months of age. It seems boring, but it is safer as it may preclude the development of allergies. If family and physician pressure breaks you down, at least use the least allergenic foods: rice, yellow vegetables, bananas, applesauce, papaya, barley, oats. No sugar or puddings. Freshly made and puréed fruits and vegetables are the most nutritious, but don't salt or sugar them. A good first step might be to start at eight months with a mashed banana with some brewer's yeast powder sprinkled on it. Smile as you push it in. Begin with a pinch and build up depending on gas.

Try to follow the principle of the four-day rotation diet. Do not offer the same food more frequently than every four days. Be sure to wait until the baby is over twelve months old to start the more common allergenic foods: wheat, eggs, citrus, and corn.

The real reason for starting solids early is to prevent the development of the milk anemia so common years ago. But it does not happen in breast-fed babies whose mothers are well-nourished, so these babies can wait until they are well over a year old to begin taking solids. This delay can further prevent the development of allergies and infections. When the baby is grabbing food off the parents' plates, it is probably time to let the child have table food.

Babies on the bottle have a problem. They need the solids, but they are already getting an allergic load because of the ingestion of cow's milk. For them, it is very important to start solids slowly and in rotation. Many parents wisely elect to stay on a formula but to use one that has iron added. They will begin the solids closer to eleven or twelve months of age, when the intestinal tract is more mature and able to cope with food.

At the first sign of a cold, allergy, rash, fussiness, wakefulness—anything out of the ordinary—stop whatever you have started and add the appropriate nutrients (usually the stress formula: vitamin C, calcium, and B complex). The symptoms are a clue that you have stressed the baby's body, and early remedial action may preclude fixed or chronic problems.

Fluoride should be given at the 0.25 mg-per-day

dose in the first year as it does toughen the unerupted teeth. I believe it prudent to give it along with some form of calcium and magnesium (cal-mag or dolomite). There is no doubt that it works; fluoridation is not a Communist plot.

The eight- to twelve-month-old often cries on separation from the mother. If he cries for two hours and gets hysterical and vomits on the babysitter, it could indicate a dysperception. Extra B complex (brewer's yeast) and calcium (dolomite) might allow him to handle these little frustrations with equanimity. Some calcium about two hours before separation time would be smart.

| Symptom or sign | Could lead to or may suggest: | Possible method of control: |
|---|---|---|
| Cold, hay fever, watery nasal discharge | Ear infection, bronchitis, recent milk change | Stop cow's milk, try goat or soy, increase vitamin C; remove cat, dog, feathers, wool |
| Green or yellow nasal discharge | Secondary infection following cold, hay fever, milk allergy, allergy to own bacteria | Change milk, control allergens, add vitamin C, try bacteria vaccine |
| Redness about anus or diaper area | Food allergy (citrus, tomato, peaches, wheat, egg) | Change diet |
| Boys: blood in urine, cries on urinating, ammonia smell | Sore just inside urethral opening | Vitamin C—100 to 300 mg at bedtime to acidify urine; add vinegar to diapers |
| Fever | Usually a virus. If aspirin (1 gr/10 lbs.) helps in 1 1/2 hours to bring down fever and infant can sit and smile, OK to wait | Use 100 to 500 mg of vitamin C every hour. Infant should be improving in twelve hours; if not, see the doctor |

| Symptom or sign | Could lead to or may suggest: | Possible method of control: |
|---|---|---|
| Fever following DPT shots | Convulsions, hurts to nervous system (rare) | Use C, D, and calcium before and after next shot |
| Fever and irritability with teething | Secondary infection, touchy child | Use C, B, and calcium during teething time |
| Loves to suck and rock | Sensitive child | Calcium, magnesium |
| Insomnia—cannot fall asleep | Sensitive, overstimulated, food allergy | Calcium, $B_6$, magnesium; hot relaxing bath; change diet |
| Insomnia—awakens often after falling asleep | Food allergy, urine burns skin | Change diet, zinc oxide or A and D ointment; extra vitamin C orally; protein at bedtime |

## Questions and Answers

**Q. When should I switch the baby from formula to homogenized pasteurized milk like we drink?**

**A.** The answer might be determined by the incidence of allergies in your family, the tendency to constipation, and the stresses you noted during your pregnancy. It might be better to introduce homogenized pasteurized milk in a cup at eight to ten months and keep the formula in the bottle. But at the first sign of a cold or ear trouble, stop the milk completely and wait at least a year or, for some, five to ten *years* before reintroducing it.

**Q. When are solids supposed to be started?**

**A.** Apparently we doctors had parents begin solids much too early. The infant's intestines could not digest foods completely, and some allergies developed which continued for a lifetime. Babies do become anemic if they are getting cow's milk alone, so a compromise is wise. Begin solids for a bottle-fed baby at about eight or nine months. Rice is usually safe. Use it once every four days. Then every month add a new food from the safe list: barley, applesauce, pears, yellow vegetables, lamb, veal, chicken.

Breast-fed babies do not become anemic if the mother is on a superior diet. Usually at ten to fourteen months the baby begins to grab food off the parents' plates. Try to aim for a no-sugar, no-white-flour diet and make some attempt to rotate the food choices. If solids are allowed first, the child will automatically adjust the milk intake to his needs. Milk is usually considered a bonus food after one year of age.

**Q. How do you get enough calcium into a one-year-old who won't drink milk?**

A. Studies have shown that we all lose 800 to 1000 mg of calcium a day; if it is not replaced, the body may respond with insomnia, muscle cramps, irritability, allergies, and clotting defects. It takes some time for the teeth and bones to demineralize. Vitamin D helps pick up the calcium and deposit it in the bones.

Dairy products are the best way to get calcium into the body, but absorption may be less than adequate because of defective intestinal enzyme production (not enough vitamin B), not enough stomach acid (vitamin C helps absorption of most minerals), or a milk allergy (try goat's milk).

Dolomite, bone meal, or oystershell calcium can be stirred into other foods. Sesame seeds, green leafy vegetables, and herbs will help get the proper amount in. Some people can eat cheese but cannot touch milk.

**Q. Is it normal for a one-year-old to lose interest in food almost completely?**

A. This usually means that the child is filling up on

milk. Sometimes there is a milk anemia and an iron tonic is necessary; a check-up and a blood test for anemia would be worthwhile. It is better to offer the solids first and let the child decide how much milk to consume afterward. Remember, no sugar.

Q. **My one-year-old son craves starches (crackers, bread, and cereal) although I made all my own baby food and use no sugar. What happened?**

A. It may be some genetic tendency or even an allergy to wheat. You may have to watch him carefully and try to allow the starches only every four days. He may have to fight a weight problem all his life. You must try to teach him to eat every two or three hours so he will never get overly hungry.

Q. **My ten-month-old is now afraid of strangers, seems easily frightened and screams when put to bed. Is he spoiled? What have we done?**

A. This separation anxiety is fairly normal at this age. It's as if the child glanced down, realized his umbilical cord was cut, and panicked. But why don't all children do this to the same extent? Can genetics explain this? Good nutrition might allow them to advance through growing phases more comfortably.

Search for food allergies—usually milk. Try extra calcium (200 to 500 mg per day) and see if the child can handle stress better. B vitamins, especially $B_6$ and pantothenic acid, may help the child say "Who cares?" or "I'm OK."

# Toddler 6
# to Six Years

After the first birthday most babies have settled down to three or four meals a day and two to four breast or bottle feedings. During this period, they gain about a pound every three months. Milk has become less important, so it makes sense to give the solids first and let the baby decide—depending on his internal control signals—how much milk is to be consumed after the solids are in.

If weaning to the cup seems important, a different-tasting fluid in the cup is usually accepted more easily. Many use 2 percent milk in the cup while continuing breast milk or formula in the bottle. A bottle-fed baby who rejects solids may be anemic; check the blood. A good general rule: If parents and siblings are feeding themselves, the baby will eventually imitate that action. Monkey see; monkey do.

Every morsel that goes in must be a nourishing food. Their bones, brains, teeth, and tissues need the best you can provide. No sugar in the house. No white flour in the house. No packaged foods. No processed foods. Dentists say children don't chew enough, and the underdeveloped jaws of adults reflect the habit of drinking juices. Let them drink the water—distilled is best. If the child must have a bottle for nap or bedtime, use water. The tooth destruction that occurs when children are allowed to hold a bottle (or breast) in their mouths all night makes pedodontists shudder. This need to suck before sleep may be due to a calcium or magnesium deficiency.

The reason you must feed only nutritious foods and stall off the introduction of the seductive, habit-forming sweets is because of the eating habits of the two- or three-year-old. A number of things happen simultaneously. They are cutting molars, they are gaining only two pounds in a year, they may be practicing noncompliance in preparation for adolescence, and they have found that not eating and whining can be a weapon to frustrate their mothers.

If they would eat, they would feel better, and if they felt better, they would eat better. Then once they don't eat, zinc and iron and B complex vitamins may be reduced, and deficiencies in these nutrients usually wreck what appetite they had. Anemic people often don't eat the foods that would correct the anemia. (Zinc deficiency will frequently affect the taste buds, making food taste terrible [dysgeusia].)

Parents may make the mistake of offering puddings, custards, and ice cream dishes just so the child will eat *something*. This compounds the problem, since most sweet-tasting foods are deficient in the very vitamins and minerals we are trying to get children to eat.

The best approach is to take all pressure off (don't push for toilet training or perfect manners), have only nutritious snacks around (if molars are not well developed, use nut butters and not nuts and seeds—aspiration danger), and make mealtimes as stressless as possible. Big servings are usually discouraging, and if you wait six hours between meals the child is having a low-blood-sugar fit or has gone into acidosis and you are dealing with a gorilla.

If a child can get up and walk around, he or she is not too sick, and if laughs and smiles are more frequent than cries and frowns, you are doing OK.

Sample day's diet for the two- to three-year-old:

| | |
|---|---|
| *Breakfast* | 2 T. whole-grain cereal made sweet with natural applesauce or raisins. 1 T. of natural peanut butter would enhance the protein quality. 2 oz. 2 percent milk. |
| *Snack* | 1-inch cube of cheese, one section of fruit, 2 oz. unsweetened juice. |
| *Lunch* | Small meatball, five pieces small steamed carrots, 2 oz. 2 percent milk. |
| *Snack* | Natural peanut butter on half slice whole wheat bread, 2 oz. unsweetened juice. |
| *Supper* | One small broiled chicken thigh, six peas, one eighth small boiled potato, 2 oz. 2 percent milk, fruit for dessert. |

Vitamin C powder can be added to the juices, brewer's yeast can be added to the nut butters, and dolomite can be put in some appropriate food at supper to ensure proper mineral intake and that bedtime will be relaxed and pleasant. Use kelp powder and sea salt instead of table salt.

By this age parents should be able to figure out by trial and error what works for their child: what foods to avoid; what infections and allergies the child is susceptible to; and the general pattern of eating, sleeping, playing, and staring at things. He should be laughing more than crying. He should be a joy, the family pride.

It is often difficult to decide if a toddler's behavior or symptoms are normal for the age, normal considering this particular child's genetic background, or whether the antics are a cry for help. A temper tantrum is about as normal as wetting the diaper, but what if the screaming and floor-pounding go on too long? And what is too long? If he still has them at age three, that's too long. If each frustration leads to a breath-holding spell and that leads to a convulsion, it *has* to mean this child's nervous system is too sensitive.

*The fifteen-month-old is usually at the peak of his temper-tantrum career.* The ones who extend this interminably may have been rewarded or reinforced by some attention they got, but many children continue because they don't feel good and are hoping, I guess, that we will finally figure out that they are anemic, have worms, are allergic to some food, or need extra calcium, zinc, or B complex vitamins. If a tantrum goes on and on to breath-holding, turning blue, eyes rolling up, falling over, and even having a convulsion, the child is really asking for help. Parents and doctors feel reassured if a brainwave test is normal, but breath-holding spells are not epilepsy.

*Treatment:* Calcium, magnesium, B$_6$, and possibly manganese would be appropriate. No sugar or white flour products and maybe a trial of no milk for a month would put a stop to them.

*Ear infections, snoring, zonking, runny nose (usually without sneezing or rubbing), throat-clearing, mouth breathing, headaches and stomachaches, pallor (not related to anemia), and dark-colored or puffy lower lids all combine to indicate an allergy—usually to milk, but wheat and eggs can do it.*

*Treatment:* All dairy products and, of course, sugar and white flour must be stopped for at least three weeks. Because the main source of calcium is gone, bone meal, dolomite, or calcium from oystershells or lactate must be substituted. It is odd that many of these children can drink raw milk with impunity, suggesting that the homogenization, pasteurization, or addition of irradiated ergosterol is the problem. But after a period of rest the body may be able to tolerate some milk again. Every fourth day for milk might be a suitable compromise.

Since this is an allergy, it would be prudent to increase the nutrients that help the adrenals. If the "milk allergy" is associated with some rhythmical activity, it suggests that the milk allergy is affecting the intestinal absorption of calcium and magnesium.

Many children with milk allergies have come from mothers who had stress during the pregnancy and were unable to nurse, the one thing that could have prevented it all.

*Sneezing, congestion, snorting, wheezing, spitting up phlegm* at various times and places are the clues that the victim is allergic to something—usually an inhalant. The allergy may be a buildup of many small allergies, none of which by themselves would be strong enough to cause trouble but collectively exhaust the adrenal glands. Many people find their allergies are minimal if they lay off sugar and white flour, which when eaten by these people cause enough biochemical stress to require cortisol secretion from the adrenals. A child may be able to sleep with the cat and a feather pillow if she does not drink milk but may have the cat, the pillow, and the milk when school (a stress) is out and the grass pollens are not blowing.

If the allergy is worse in the morning, something in the bed or room is usually responsible. Cortisol secretion is supposed to be at its peak at this time, so some of the adrenal-gland support nutrients would be appropriate at bedtime.

*Treatment:* Increase vitamin C intake as the allergies increase; the worse the allergy the more vitamin C should be consumed. The end point would be sloppy bowel movements. Pantothenic acid and $B_6$ are helpful in controlling allergies. Calcium (1000 mg per day) helps with the stress of allergies. Some take a long-acting vitamin C at bedtime and sneeze less in the morning.

*The two-year-old has usually discovered what activity bothers his parents most.* Sucking, rocking, banging, awakening at night, walking on his heels, singing off key, and pulling knobs off the TV are all reasonably tolerated by the parents until this age group adds the refinements of whining and not eating. We all seem to intuit that if the child would eat better, he would feel better and stop whining, but he won't stop whining long enough to eat. Cutting three-year molars is a stress. The pressures of toilet training are a stress. If the nutrition was barely adequate before, the appetite loss and stress related to just being two often puts the child at such a level of vulnerability that he will be hyperactive, allergic, or susceptible to infections.

*Treatment:* Prevention is always the best treatment. Every morsel should be as nourishing as possible. If the child has become used to sweets, he may go hungry when served turnip greens and beans. When he first began to eat solids at about one year of age, he should have been getting used to brewer's yeast, wheat germ, and kelp. He must be allowed to nibble; small amounts of fruits and vegetables, legumes, peanut butter, egg, and cheese should be around so he can eat almost constantly. Don't expect him to eat three big meals a day. By the time the meal comes around, his falling blood sugar may make him so miserable he can only be crabby and petulant; he doesn't know he is supposed to eat.

*About 10 percent of two- through six-year-olds act as if they are being sent to the gallows.* He may sit at the edge of the pool or the dancing class with his thumb in his mouth and his heart racing, hoping no one will notice him. He is scared to death. It may be that his space bubble is constricted; his world is collapsing. His pulse rate may be rapid (check it) because of the adrenalin flowing as a result of falling blood sugar from something he ate. He may act scared because of the adrenalin; it does not have to mean he has adrenalin because he is scared. But because he happened to secrete adrenalin simultaneously with attendance at one of these classes, he will be reminded each time he goes. He felt afraid once, and his memory tells him that this is the place where he was uncomfortable before.

*Treatment:* Any new situation can be faced with aplomb if the blood sugar can be maintained at an even level. If blood sugar falls because of a quick carbohydrate meal simultaneous with stress, the coping part of the brain will malfunction and stress will be handled by the animal brain with depression, fear, aches, asthma, or some psychosomatic response. Everyone should be fortified with a protein snack before anything even remotely stressful: first day of school or lessons or party, seeing the doctor or dentist, going to bed (a stress for many children), or a dancing class. A rough evaluation of the internal metabolism could be made by testing the pulse (60 to 70 best) and the pH of saliva with litmus paper (6.5 to 7.0 best).

We expect a certain amount of noncompliance from our children, but many children act out their frustrations because they simply do not feel well. "Find something wrong with this child!" is the clenched-teeth demand by many parents of the eighteen-month- to four-year-old. The parents had hoped an ear infection, or anemia, or even a molar pushing through could be found to explain the surly behavior.

"Something you're doing is wrong" is the implied suggestion from the doctor and seconded by the in-laws. How depressing. How maddening. You love the child, but it would be nice if you could like him also.

| Symptom or sign | Could lead to or may suggest: | Possible way to alleviate: |
|---|---|---|
| Won't eat good food | Anemia, hypoglycemia, bad taste | Needs iron, B vitamins, zinc, better cooking |
| Jekyll-and-Hyde mood swings, ups and downs | Hypoglycemia, food allergy | Nibble, B vitamins, calcium |
| Insomnia, or Won't fall asleep } | Too much stimulation | Hot bath, calcium, Tryptophan, stop sugar |
| Awakens in night | Hypoglycemia, food allergy | Change diet |
| Aggressive, surly, mean, hits, fights, chip on shoulder, noncompliant | Cutting teeth, low blood sugar, feels stressed by home, depression, food allergy, heavy metal poisoning, abnormal brainwaves | Calcium, magnesium, B vitamins, stop sugar, search for food allergy, hair test for heavy metal poisoning. |
| Sick too much | Stress, teeth, food allergy (milk), see your doctor | Increase vitamin C until loose BM; use rutin, bioflavenoids, vitamin A; stop sugar |
| Allergies, asthma, hay fever, hives | Exhausted adrenal glands | Vitamin C to tolerance, pantothenic acid, $B_6$, calcium, zinc, vitamin A |
| Shy, frightened, avoids eye contact, rocks, sucks, twists, is ticklish | Fears, missing a lot of fun in life | Calcium, B vitamins, $B_6$, $B_3$, manganese, magnesium |

## Questions and Answers

Q. Why do babies and children have to rock themselves to sleep on hands and knees?

**A.** They feel more comfortable or they wouldn't do it. It does not have to mean they are insecure. They may be suppressing uncomfortable stimuli from their intestines, skin, or muscles. Try some calcium. Change the diet; maybe an allergy is doing it.

**Q. I have a four-year-old who sits and picks at dinner for two hours. She does not enjoy eating. She sucks her thumb while holding onto a ripped, rotten security blanket.**

**A.** Get a good medical checkup to make sure she is not sick or anemic. An iron tonic with B vitamins may help. Some who do not like the taste of food are low in zinc. Don't make an issue of it. Try to put small amounts of food on her plate so she won't be discouraged. (Example: one cube of meat or cheese, eight peas and a quarter of a boiled potato, two ounces of milk, and sixteen grapes for dessert.) Have nuts and seeds in bowls about the house and raw vegetables and fruit in the refrigerator. Let her nibble.

**Q. Why do two- to four-year-olds have so many fears—bugs, darkness, and monsters?**

**A.** Most children love the excitement and the flow of adrenalin that comes with scary things. But they want the excitement in the sweet security of their family. We must be reassuring and comforting. Leave lights on.

Some children become frightened of some area, person, or thing because they happened to be hit with a blast of adrenalin when they were nearby. A child who ate a sugary breakfast may suffer a rapid heart and a feeling of fright simultaneously with stepping in the door of nursery school. When blood sugar falls, adrenalin comes into the circulation and makes the child think the reaction was to the school. You may never get him back into that school because of his anxiety association.

**Q. My two-and-a-half-year-old daughter falls asleep after masturbating. In the last few months since potty**

training, she keeps her hands in her underpants. Do we get hysterical?

A. Keep your cool. Masturbation is such a common phenomenon in the two- to six-year-old and the adolescent (and adult) that if it doesn't happen we wonder what is wrong. The child should get the message that it is OK, but not in public as "people do not understand."

Frequently the child's attention is drawn to the area because of an itch. Take a look. The redness in the area is more likely due to a food allergy (milk, wheat, citrus, tomato, chocolate) than to friction. Is orange juice an aphrodisiac, too? (See pages 111 to 112.)

Q. How do you deal with a two-year-old saying "mine" and not letting anyone near his toys?

A. A real dog in the manger. Usually nursery schools don't allow children under three to enter because of this selfish, unable-to-share attitude. But the fact that he is so uncompromising suggests he does not feel good. Try the diet changes. Treat him for worms and add extra calcium and B vitamins. By the time you figure it out, he will be in some other phase.

Q. How do you get a two-year-old away from the bottle with as little trauma as possible?

A. It is important to forbid sugary drinks because the teeth may rot. Be slow. Gradually replace the milk with water, then gradually reduce the amount of water until the child is sucking an empty bottle, then just the nipple. The child knows when he or she does not need to suck any more. This whole process may take months or years. If you do it too rapidly, the child becomes suspicious that he is being cheated and may throw the rejected bottle at you. Calcium may help.

Q. Our five-year-old daughter has been on a milk- and gluten-free diet since she was eight months old. She still gets ear infections with each cold. How come? She takes vitamin C and bioflavenoids daily.

A. She may need more vitamin C. Increase the dose daily until she gets some looseness in her bowls, then cut back. When she gets a cold, give that daily dose hourly. Vitamin A may be necessary (up to 20,000 to 30,000 units per day for thirty days). She may be allergic to some other food (corn, potatoes, eggs) that you thought was safe. An inhalant (feathers, mold, cat, dog, wool) could trigger it. She may need her adenoids out. The previous infections may have caused them to swell and surgery may be necessary now. Nutrition may not shrink them. She may be allergic to her own bacteria.

Q. My sixteen-month-old continually eats paper, whether hungry or not. Is she missing something?

A. Probably she is calling out to you that she is missing some vitamin or mineral. (She also can get a heavy metal poisoning from the lead or other metals in the ink.) Eating nonfoods is called pica and usually represents an anemia due to iron deficiency. But she may need calcium, zinc, magnesium, or the B vitamins. Experiment after a blood test for anemia and iron storage. A hair test, which reveals relative amounts of minerals stored in the hair, may pinpoint a deficiency or an overload.

Q. How can a grandmother encourage (or insist) that the diet of her hyperactive grandchild be altered without offending her daughter-in-law?

A. Usually it's the mother requesting aid in dealing with the grandmother. ("Sugar is love, dearie; one cookie won't hurt.") You could try something tangential like "I noticed the other day when I took Eddie shopping and he insisted on a cola drink, he seemed virtually to explode. Have you noticed anything like that? Is it an allergy?" Try to get her on your side with this one: "You know, Charlie (my son, your husband) was a lot like Eddie when he was a youngster. I had to feed him whole-grain, nourishing cereal every morning or he would be all over the classroom." Keep at it, at least by example; you'll get the message across.

Q. My five-year-old son frequently appears in the late afternoon demanding "something sweet." When offered some fruit he replies "I want some real sugar, like cookies." Is this hypoglycemic behavior?

A. Probably. The craving for very sugary sweets comes from the eating of very sugary sweets. The blood sugar rises and falls rapidly, and the speed of its plunge sets up a craving that cannot be ignored. The lack of proper energy at the neocortical level may interrupt any good intentions or veto previous promises, as in an alcoholic. It would be wise not to have any sweets around a house where people have these cravings. They should nibble on nuts, seeds, cheese, and fruit. The B complex vitamins, especially $B_3$, seem to keep the blood sugar from dropping too low.

A most important action is to change the lunch and snacks he must be getting at kindergarten.

Q. We got a sandbox for our two-year-old, and although he does play in it, he loves to eat it. His stools are often gritty. Is this bad?

A. Not usually, unless the cats are using it as a litter box. He may just be curious, but it could also mean pica. Eating nonfoods is supposed to be a sign of a mineral deficiency. Eating dirt may mean the person is low in iron (or zinc or copper). Eating sand suggests he is searching for calcium, magnesium, or phosphorus. Try oyster shell calcium and send him out again.

Q. How early do you recommend allergy tests on children?

A. Most allergists feel that testing is not valid until the child is over eighteen months of age, and then skin tests are not a reliable method of determining food allergies. Because cow's milk is such a common allergen and the infant is consuming such a load of it, everything from the cow should be discontinued if an allergy is suspected. Allergies cannot do everything, but they can cause anything from ear infections, asthma, rashes, gas, arthritis, and crabbiness to insomnia. It takes about a month off dairy products to be sure they are the villain.

Try to aim for the four-day rotation diet, and if inhalants are suspected, clean out the child's sleeping room, use electric heat, foam-rubber toys, and dump the cat. Assuming the adrenal glands are exhausted, use the support system to help them make their own cortisol.

**Q. What could cause bad breath in a child?**

**A.** Or anyone. The most likely problem is some food fermenting in the intestines. The putrid matter is absorbed into the bloodstream, is not filtered out sufficiently by the liver, gets to the lungs, and is exhaled. If the malodor is present every day, it would suggest that a food eaten every day is not digested properly. Possibly an allergy. Don't forget chronically infected tonsils, postnasal drip, and odd items shoved up the nostrils and forgotten. Rotten teeth are a possibility, or even teeth pushing through the gums. Acidosis from fluctuations of blood sugar might give a different odor. Extra vitamins (expecially B, C, and E) might help the body detoxify the poisons.

**Q. My eighteen-month-old has had eczema since age three months. He's on soybean formula. Could I try goat's milk?**

**A.** He might do better on a rotation diet: goat's milk on Monday, soy on Tuesday, meat milk on Wednesday, and so on. Assume he has exhausted adrenals and his family disease showed up. Another child might have asthma or ear infections. At least be slow on the introduction of solids and try to crowd a lot of C, $B_6$, pantothenic acid, calcium, and zinc into him. It should all help him "outgrow" it faster.

**Q. My four-year-old takes phenobarbital because**

he has had three febrile seizures. How can his diet be altered to stop the seizures?

A. First, don't let him get sick again; build up his immune systems with vitamin C and vitamin A. Calcium, magnesium, manganese, and $B_6$ all have a calming effect on the nervous system. He should have a nibbling diet—small amounts frequently. Taper him off the phenobarbital over the next three to six months. He will have outgrown the seizure tendency by then anyway. Check with your doctor.

Q. Other than eggs, cheese, and peanut butter, what do you suggest feeding a thirteen-month-old who refuses everything else except bread?

A. Actually, that's a pretty good diet. Dealing with children and their eating habits is a compromise between the cheerful intake of all the proper nutrients and the forceful feeding of the stubborn beast. If a checkup reveals no pathology and no anemia, at least try a few sneaky things like brewer's yeast (a smidgeon to start) and kelp in the peanut butter. Throw things on the floor and say "Don't eat that." It works for one day. (And try the recipes in this book.)

Q. I know if my three-year-old would eat better, he would feel better, and if he felt better, he would eat better. How is it done?

A. Try the recipes. Help him with his own vegetable patch; if he grows it, he might eat it. Help *him* steam the veggies. Make carrot cake or squash cake with a smidgeon of honey. Is there a broccoli cake? He can become deficient in zinc, which may further distort his touchy taste buds. Don't load up his plate; ten peas on a coffee saucer may be a big dinner.

If he smiles more than he frowns, he'll make it.

Q. What would cause a stomachache in a hyper child? Sometimes it ends in vomiting.

A. We were trained to believe that this type of

response is psychogenic. Most hyper kids overreact to their environment, so the setup is right. But we also know that low blood sugar can force the body to use fat for energy and acidosis may result; acidosis is associated with nausea and vomiting. (See page 212 for a more detailed explanation.) If there is migraine in the family and you find acetone in his urine in the morning, he probably has cyclic vomiting. His metabolism will not allow him to use glycogen stored in the liver and he burns fat.

Change his diet (could there be an allergy?) and make sure he gets some protein every night. That ice cream at bedtime might be doing it.

**Q. How old does a child have to be to benefit from spanking?**

**A.** Children need discipline and rules, but we hope to avoid physical punishment—which, in general, promotes the idea that violence is an acceptable activity. The battered child may grow to batter his children. A swat on the bare bottom usually gets a child's attention if he seems out of control, but if a child seems continually to "ask" for it by unacceptable behavior, parents must back off and decide if their rules are unrealistic (for instance, expecting toilet training at one year of age) or whether the child is trying to communicate that he doesn't feel good. Jekyll-and-Hyde behavior, especially, is the clue that a nutrition defect probably exists. Rewarding good, socially approved behavior is the best way to build in a conscience that is not too restrictive when the child becomes an adult.

Spankings are usually not begun until the gregarious child begins to cruise at twelve to eighteen months. Early discipline should be confined to alerting the child to danger. It is OK to get excited when he or she is running into a busy street.

**Q. I am a pediatrician and agree with much of what you say. I have noted, however, that many of the children**

develop their hyperactive symptoms and noncompliant behavior within a few minutes after ingesting sugar. This suggests an allergic response, as a quick carbohydrate would elevate the blood sugar—at least for a while.

**A.** You are right, but my understanding is that several mechanisms may be operating simultaneously. In some children the blood sugar will rise for twenty to sixty minutes and then plummet. In others the pancreas is so sensitive that the insulin knocks down the blood sugar within minutes. In a third group the blood sugar bounces up and down so fast that acidosis sets in, and this causes the adverse reaction. (Litmus-paper testing of the salivary pH should be diagnostic.) A cerebral allergy (a hive on the brain?) might be the explanation. It is known that histamine release (one of the allergy mediators) will cause restless behavior. It is beyond me why many doctors cannot believe this emotional lability is diet-induced.

# Six Years Old 7
## to Puberty

Exuberance and enthusiasm about the world and its creatures characterize most growing children. Educational dysfunction should be detected early so remediation can be effected before the child develops negative attitudes about school or a bad self-image. No child should go to school without his brain; no teacher should have to teach a child who did not bring his brain to school. Teachers are becoming clever enough to ask children what they had for breakfast, especially those who are pale, tired, spacey, restless, or inconsistent in their performance. Parents should feed their children a protein, fruit, or vegetable snack as soon as they come home from school. Wait twenty minutes and *then* ask "How did it go in school today?" Checking the salivary pH may help explain dirty looks, obscene gestures, foul language, and even clumsy actions.

The six-year-old–to–puberty age group is still heavily dependent upon parents for a support system. Once adolescence is reached our children tend to look for peer group acceptance. If we want to direct them into a happy,

71

productive life, these years may be the only chance we
have. With our help they can develop good health habits of
eating and living. Doctors, dentists, teachers, and ministers
("The body is the temple of the soul") can play a significant
role in influencing our children. We may have to remind
these leaders that they do wield considerable clout. I have
had mothers slip me notes: "Tell him to eat his spinach." I
do, and many times he will. A child may brush her teeth for
the dentist but not for her parents.

Children in the classroom set up their pecking order
despite our and the teachers' efforts to civilize the
little animals. Winners and losers take their places in this
hierarchy, and those at the bottom end are more likely the
hyperactive, the klutzy, the oddballs, the absentees, and
the sickly weaklings. Before they get a label that may last
for a lifetime and before they develop a bad self-image, we
have to intervene somehow. One way is to supply optimum
nutrition so the appropriate part of the brain is functioning
when called upon to think.

| Symptoms and signs | What it means or could lead to: | What may help: |
| --- | --- | --- |
| Insomnia | Falling blood sugar and adrenal release, pinworms, low minerals, food allergy | Protein at bedtime, antihistamines; add calcium, magnesium, zinc, manganese |
| Paleness, tiredness, circles under eyes, aches (stomach and head) | Food allergy, usually milk; check for anemia | Change diet, add vitamin C and B complex |
| Loves sweets, poor school performance | Hypoglycemia, exhaustion, depression, hyperactivity | No sugar, no junk; add B vitamins, protein, nuts, seeds, vegetable diet |

| Symptoms and signs | What it means or could lead to: | What may help: |
| --- | --- | --- |
| Had tonsils and adenoids out, now craves milk, jiggles foot up and down | Milk allergy, low body calcium, other allergies or hyperactivity | Calcium; stop milk or whatever food is being craved |
| Won't or cannot sit in A.M. | Low blood sugar, eating wrong food the night before, maybe in acidosis in A.M.; without breakfast may not function in school | Stop sugar; add protein at bedtime, compromise: eat two almonds every 30 minutes in A.M. |

From six to ten years of age the appetite is fairly even, and although they have strong likes and dislikes, most children get a variety of foods. The teachers, relatives, and parents of playmates can serve as great reinforcers in your attempt to keep junk out of your child for as long as possible. Of course, the parents must stop eating non-nourishing foods, also. An exercise program is a must. No smoking is allowed (child or adult).

Growing their own vegetables, planning a week's menus, cooking a meal for the parents will all help to fix into children's brains that we have to eat good food. Sometimes we compromise: "I notice you didn't get all your calcium requirements today. How do you suggest we do that?" A couple of calcium tablets at bedtime might be the answer. Or "I know you don't like these parsnips. Eat the chicken for your protein and take three kelp tablets. But what do we do for your fiber requirements?" The child responds with "I'll chew up some bran with my cereal in the morning." "Good thinking."

But what do we do about Halloween, Easter, birthday parties, and well-meaning friends who feel "sugar is love"? Relatives think these children are deprived and sneak candy to them.

The devil's tempting sweets are omnipresent, and your child will become a victim of his own taste buds and biochemistry. Logic does not work—especially if you are talking to the child's lower animal brain. Use the pre-party protein plan (some protein [about two tablespoons], vitamin C [1000 mg], B complex [50 mg of each], and 500 mg of calcium ingested about a half hour before the event keeps the blood sugar even and prevents an allergic reaction to some party foods. Also makes one a better guest), and when he arrives home make sure he gets some postparty stress antidote (B complex, vitamin C, and calcium). This also can prevent hangovers for adults.

Calcium and magnesium deficiencies are common in our country. This fact helps to explain the restlessness and insomnia so often reported. Part of the defect is explained by the consumption of an enormous amount of soft drinks in place of milk; some of the fault has to be due to the use of chocolate milk and inadequate intestinal absorption. A lot of milk is going down into the stomach, but some factor is inhibiting its uptake into the system.

Parents should at least be aware that there could be a problem, especially in the children who seem to have outgrown their milk allergies. The allergy could move to another organ. It would be worthwhile to sit down with a table of food values and a list of what foods actually were swallowed by your child in any week. See if the child is close to the recommended daily allowances. These RDAs are only for survival, but they are a start:

Vitamin A—5000 units
Vitamin D—500 units
Vitamin C—60–100 mg
B complex—2–30 of the various Bs
Zinc—15 mg

Calcium—1000 mg
Magnesium—500 mg
Fluoride—1 mg
Vitamin E—100 units

If you are not sure, at least get a supplement down that gets close to these values. Then read your child's body and figure out what extra supplements the child needs because he or she is unique. After a month of the supplements, you may have lifted your child (and yourself) out of a self-perpetuating nutritional hole. Then, by using the recipes in this book specifically designed to supply those needed supplements, you may be able to maintain the child in optimum health.

*One of the most disturbing observations I made in my pediatric practice was the difference in susceptibility to infection and allergies in children*—how some with indifferent care might sneeze once a year. Genetic factors, stresses during the pregnancy, plus a difficult delivery and inadequate nursing seem to be precursors of these children's unhealthiness.

*Treatment:* Now that we know that enzymes are responsible for the manufacture of immune substances and the integrity of white cells and that these enzymes are maintained by adequate amounts of vitamin C and B, we should have the skill and foresight to use nutrients when we know someone has been exposed to an illness or it is the flu season.

The second or third case of chickenpox in a family is usually more severe, as if the virus has increased in virulence. It is prudent to increase the daily vitamin C dose to an amount that loosens the bowels slightly. Fruit juices, peppers, onions—all laced with vitamin C—should increase the amount of intracellular interferon and reduce the severity of chickenpox, cold, flu, mono—whatever the virus. This also works in anticipation of DPT and measles shots.

Allergic people usually are more susceptible to superimposed infections. If allergies are seasonal, the nutrients that help the adrenal glands should be increased before the troublesome season. If one is required to eat a food that causes symptoms, a protective protein feeding plus extra calcium (500 to 1000 mg), vitamin C (1000 to 2000 mg), and vitamin $B_6$ (500 mg) should keep the reaction to the allergen at a minimum.

It is estimated that 80 percent of those with food allergies have related problems with blood-sugar fluctuations. We know that a rapid fall of blood sugar will stimulate the adrenals to secrete more cortisol. Then, with the adrenals exhausted, an allergy will surface. If the food to which the victim is allergic is consumed, the blood sugar begins to fluctuate, further exhausting the depleted adrenals. The victim may only recognize an "all-gone feeling," stuffiness, gas, tiredness, and a craving for quick carbohydrates. His body may be craving the sweets Mother Nature has produced in fruits, but he may not be able to satisfy this except with sugary quick carbohydrates, devoid of C and B. Blood sugar rises and falls, cortisol is depleted, allergies become manifest or a sickness occurs.

### Questions and Answers

**Q. What should a parent do about a ten-year-old bedwetter? I've ignored it until now, but something has to be done. The doctor says there is nothing physically wrong. I worry about his feelings about himself.**

**A.** Boys are supposed to outgrow this distressing problem by age five or so (girls by age four). Deep sleep may allow the bladder to empty automatically. (Give some protein, nuts, seeds, or other long-term energy source at bedtime.) An allergy may trigger the problem. (Try the four-day rotation diet or stop milk, wheat, or whatever is being eaten daily.) Magnesium may allow the bladder to stretch and hold more urine.

Research has revealed that many bedwetters have an abnormal sleep-cycle pattern, and a training program with a light and bells connected to a screen in the bed can change this back to normal. A bedwetting device is available at Sears.

**Q. My eight-year-old daughter is so shy it hurts. She's missing a lot of fun in her life. Every day has a new concern: "What if . . . ?" She still sucks her thumb and needs a night light. She has one friend who is shy also. Is psychiatry next?**

A. Possibly, but before that, see if you can find some biochemical reason for her withdrawal. She is telling you that the world is too close; she perceives her environment too keenly. Her adrenalin flows too easily because her brain gets too many messages; her space bubble is constricted.

You can present opportunities for social contact, but don't push her too hard or she will resent you also. You should be able to make her life more comfortable by using the no-sugar, nibbling-on-good-food diet. Stop any food she loves—especially junk. If she really craves dairy products, there may be a calcium deficiency. Stop the milk and add 1000 mg of calcium to the diet daily.

**Q. We have three children: an eleven-year-old boy, a six-year-old girl, and a boy toddler. They fight all the time. The girl especially is very aggressive, and no one can stand her.**

A. Behavior modification experts have success with the "turning your back on bad behavior" routine. It's hard to do when you are sure someone will get hurt. It's also possible that she does not feel good because of a food allergy (usually to her favorite food), or low blood sugar (eating sweets), or she is anemic, has a chronic infection eating away at her, or has pinworms.

**Q. I know my seven-year-old girl would do better in the morning if she had some nourishment in her at the moment of awakening, but she's so crabby she won't do anything I say. Do I pass the stomach tube and squirt some soup down?**

A. Sometimes the early morning noncompliance and antisocial behavior is due to low blood sugar from something eaten (or nothing eaten) at bedtime. Try a protein snack at bedtime and, of course, eliminate any sugar from the diet. A food allergy can explain the same gorilla behavior. Can you sneak in and poke some protein drink into her before she is awake? It's probably best to just get out of her way; sounds like you are dealing with her spinal cord.

**Q. A boy down the street (age about eleven) loves to sniff gasoline. He hangs around the local garage, he takes the caps off gas tanks, and I think he sniffs glue also. Is he retarded or crazy?**

A. He may be neither. But he is waving a flag; he wants some help. He is trying to dull his perception of the world, which he may find is uncomfortable. You have an obligation to inform his parents of your observations; they should seek help.

My experience with these children is that they feel they are losers. Sad people sniff petrochemicals; he feels bad about himself. The more he sniffs, the more addled he will become. Heavy users may lose brain cells, just as alcoholics do. The curiosity of that age group gets them started, then the biochemical craving perpetuates the self-destruction. They are self-destructive because the part of their brain that says "I'm a nice person" is not operative. Nutrition, good food, a lot of B vitamins, and calcium and magnesium plus a nonjudgmental, firm, kind intervention by a warm human being should turn the situation around before permanent damage occurs.

**Q. Obesity runs in my family, and my husband tends to gain easily. We have a four-year-old daughter who is 40 inches tall and weighs 40 pounds. A little chunky. Is she stuck for life?**

A. Genetic factors are present in most cases, and it sounds like she has the tendency. You have to be more watchful of her diet, exercise, and life style in general. Have no sugar or white flour in your house. She must be taught to nibble six to eight times a day at nuts, seeds, raw vegetables. Fats and starches are to be restricted—also for her father.

Don't try to make her lose; it's too tough on children. See if you can keep her from gaining more than six pounds a year—half a pound per month.

**Q. My child loves sweets, but I know they make him loud and restless. He won't eat anything that isn't sugary. How do I change? Is honey OK?**

A. Honey and fruit have fructose (along with dextrose), which is a sweet sugar but does not make the blood sugar rise so rapidly and consequently does not make the pancreas secrete insulin so rapidly. Fructose does turn into dextrose and is used for energy, so it is still a sugar. Its use promotes the idea to a child (or adult) that food must taste sweet.

You may use honey or fructose on the foods of the sweet-cravers in gradually decreasing amounts. In three months you tell your child "Sorry, the bees stopped making the stuff."

Dentists tell me that because honey sticks to the teeth so well, it is more cariogenic than table sugar.

# Adolescence 8 to Adulthood

Controlling the diet and limiting the intake of antinutrients during the six-to-twelve-year-old range is to prepare the child's body for the stressful onslaught of adolescence. Emotional, hormonal, and growth stresses plus peer pressures are so strong and compelling that even the most stable, optimally nourished child will tend to tilt.

The rates of depression, suicide, crime, acting out, running away, drug abuse, and sexual experimentation skyrocket among eleven-to-eighteen-year-olds. No one has even counted the numbers of youths with acne, headaches, growing pains, mononucleosis, gas, and bad self-image.

They grow so fast—sometimes four inches in a year—that hunger is overpowering, and once they find peace and comfort in French fries and soft drinks, they are hooked into a long-term pattern of quick carbohydrate, fat, and salt ingestion. A logical approach to initiate a diet change is nearly impossible. What thirteen-year-old listens to Mom or Dad?

"You know about tooth decay and sugar, don't you?"

"I'll brush my teeth and take fluoride."

"Don't you want to feel better when you get up in the morning?"

"Feel better for what? School? You're kidding."

"Don't you want to get rid of your headache?"

"I take aspirin."

"Don't you want to lose weight?"

"I'll go on a diet—someday."

Children at this age are exquisitely vulnerable to peer-group pressure. Some can exist and even feel good on the "in" diet of fast foods. Most young people try pot, alcohol, drugs just for a fun high: the thing to do for peer acceptance. As they experiment many find they feel good on drugs, probably because the substance suppresses some symptom of a deficiency. (Alcohol temporarily relieves the depressing symptoms of hypoglycemia.) It is difficult to stand by and watch your own child get deeper and deeper into drugs, depression, and a turned-off existence. Taking a clue from the work of Dr. Alfred Libby and Dr. Irwin Stone, it seems quite logical and simple to get extra vitamin C into these people (20 to 50 grams a day); then because they feel better they act better, and you might be able to reverse the downhill trend. Pure vitamin C is cheap and safe. The powder could be put into the youth's juice, and no one would be the wiser.

We used to say that adolescence was just a time for prayer and breath-holding. But if we can keep the youth's neocortex functioning optimally with nourishing feedings every two to four hours, we should be able to relax because the good self-image and the conscience filed away in that area will be alert and functioning.

Although all of us have been through adolescence, we only become experts in our own adolescence. When we are faced with another's adolescence (our child's, our patient's) we are often at a loss to be helpful or even understanding. Every person is unique, and it is difficult to make general rules about how to help our children or our patients through this tumultuous time. But this age group triggers more questions and anxieties than any other.

So many forces are operative on this group that it is almost impossible to ferret out which does what; give us a nice clean case of pneumonia any time. My experience with growing children is that if they can survive the pangs of emerging into adulthood with some ego intact, they will be reasonably normal as adults. But the key to that survival is based to no small degree on the events they have experienced from *conception* on. The pregnancy is the launching pad.

If a pregnant woman is low in B$_6$, she may vomit. She may not get all her nutrients and feels so punk she may not nurse her somewhat premature baby, who develops a milk allergy and suffers some hearing loss—which prevents an optimum learning experience. He is told he could do better if he would try harder. He thought he had. He gets a bad self-image; he hates himself and school. He can find others who share similar feelings. He feels gypped and cheated. All this from a lack of a vitamin? It's hard to believe, but there *have* to be better reasons than those purely psychological or sociological factors. They are too simplistic.

The turned-off adolescent may have gotten his poor self-image because he did not feel well. If he did not feel well, he may have been told to "shape up" or "you could do better."

It is easier to rear a child, show respect, offer love and give a child a sense of worth if the child has been cheerful, thoughtful, compliant, and has felt well. Laughing at his father's jokes helps too. This love and acceptance he received in childhood has to hold him through the many negatives of adolescence.

But the "I'm OK" circuit is filed in the top of the neocortex of the brain. That circuit has to be energized with good food or the owner will forget he *is* OK. We as parents, teachers, and physicians have to keep that thought alive. After all, these young punks have to take care of us someday.

| Symptoms and signs | Could lead to or may suggest: | Possible method of control: |
|---|---|---|
| Allergy | Exhausted adrenals | Vitamins and minerals, avoid allergens, stop sugar and stress |
| Arthritis | Food allergy, family tendency, stress, and exhausted adrenals | Change diet, add vitamins C, B complex, zinc, calcium, niacinamide, eliminate food allergens. |
| Depression | Ineffective brain enzymes | Avoid sugar, try mega doses of B vitamins, especially $B_{12}$ and folic acid |
| Addiction | Biochemical imbalance | Nourishing diet, counseling, vitamin C, 30 to 60 grams a day |
| Antisocial behavior | Bad self-image, poor diet | Nourishing diet, no sugar or junk; add vitamin C, B complex, and calcium |
| Obesity | Hypoglycemia | Complex carbohydrate and protein diet, B vitamins, stop milk and beef |

| Symptoms and signs | Could lead to or may suggest: | Possible method of control: |
|---|---|---|
| Schizophrenia | Biochemical fault (20 possible reasons for dysperception), copper poisoning | No milk, beef, sugar or wheat; add 3000 mg of $B_3$ and C, 500 mg of $B_6$ |
| Alcoholism | Hypoglycemia, vitamin and mineral depletion | Nibble on nourishing food; mega doses of B; magnesium, calcium, and zinc |
| Restlessness, hyperactivity | Becomes truck driver, talk show host, or criminal | Nourishing diet, no junk, B complex, especially $B_6$; calcium and magnesium help |

## Questions and Answers

Q. My niece is thirteen and has anorexia nervosa. She is bright, athletic but cannot be talked out of the crazy idea that she is fat! Five foot three and 85 pounds! She sees a psychiatrist, but so far no improvement.

A. Psychic and nutritional forces combine to make this impossible to treat with only one modality. The holistic approach helps. These people, usually girls, decide that becoming a mature person is frightening. By not eating, they feel, maturation is delayed and the responsibilities and the sexuality of womanhood will be avoided.

A combination of psychotherapy, behavior modification, and vitamin and mineral supplementation has the best chance of success.

Q. My husband is pretty healthy but loves salt, potato chips, pickles, olives, crackers, and needs them every day. He sprinkles salt on everything he eats. I worry because there is hypertension in his family. How do I get him to cut down?

A. A very common craving. It usually means he is looking for some vitamin (B complex) or mineral (usually calcium or zinc). Or his taste has been altered so that he must use extra salt to enhance the flavor of the food. It takes about a week of extra B vitamins or dolomite or kelp (which has thirty to forty trace minerals) to lose the craving.

It's better to be slow and sneaky by mixing vegetable salt, kelp, or sea salt with the table salt in gradually increasing amounts. If you do it right, your family won't notice. Extra sodium does lead, in susceptible people, to high blood pressure. Vegetarians have much less hypertension; there is very little sodium in vegetables. Beef, cheese, and milk contain a lot of sodium, so people who eat those foods should really cut back on table salt.

Q. I am a nineteen-year-old student in college and do fine after a breakfast of cereal, egg, and milk. I think and study and take notes all morning but can't keep my eyes open after lunch; I like my one o'clock class. Lunch is usually two sandwiches with cheese, peanut butter, or cold meats. What's happening?

A. If you had jelly with the peanut butter, I would say that it was an attack of hypoglycemia. But because the sandwich filler is different each day, I would tend to blame the wheat in the bread, especially if you like it. Try a bagful of raw vegetables, seeds, nuts, a piece of cheese, and an apple. You should know in just a day or two. Occasionally a 500-mg tablet of niacinamide is a good pickup.

Q. My son-in-law is a lovely, thoughtful, and almost perfect father to my grandchildren, but he will not eat vegetables. Last month he lost his sense of taste. Is there a connection?

A. Easily. We are supposed to eat a variety of foods so we get a variety of vitamins and minerals to make the body work properly. If the farmers have fertilized the soil with seaweed or a preparation containing all the trace minerals, then eating vegetables would be appropriate. He could have lost his sense of taste because he was eating poorly fertilized crops. Kelp is a good source of thirty to forty trace minerals, but extra zinc (30 to 60 mg) for a while should bring the taste buds back to optimal function.

Q. I am fourteen years old and used to have good, clear skin. Now I'm loaded with zits and am taking Erythro-mycin (R), which gives me a stomachache.

A. That is the standard treatment, but a vitamin-A derivative in the form of an acid will help to clear the skin. Some dermatologists are learning that there is a nutritional approach that will enhance their control rate. No sugar, no chocolate, no salt, no dairy products, and no beef is basic. The latter two might be added back cautiously after a month or so. You must try to nibble on raw fruits and vegetables. Go to the health store and get some zinc (like the gluconate or chelated zinc); 60 mg a day is about right. Some find vitamin A internally helps, but big doses can be toxic after a while. Check with your doctor.

Q. My eighteen-year-old nephew had two beers, was caught speeding, and ended up in jail because he assaulted the policeman who arrested him. My sister is not a perfect mother, but did she cause all that?

A. Wild, impulsive, and inappropriate behavior may be the result of falling blood sugar (beer on an empty stomach), which could allow the humane, social brain with its conscience to become unable to exert any control. The animal brain took over. The judge won't let him off, but somehow your nephew has to understand he can drink only one third of a beer and it must be accompanied by twenty almonds and some B complex. The part of the brain that is responsible for insight also disappears with a drink or two. It's like there are two people inside him. The only thing your sister did was to pass on the gene (or marry someone with it) that leads to overproduction of insulin in response to quick carbohydrate (beer).

Q. My daughter, age sixteen, is tired all the time. She is cold when others are comfortable. She is just a little overweight. The doctor did a thyroid test: normal. He said she would snap out of this when she gets a boyfriend. We may have to bring one in; she's too tired to go out and get one of her own.

A. She still may have a sluggish thyroid. A low normal for the laboratory may be an outright deficiency for her. Take her temperature orally before she gets out of bed in the morning; it should register 97.8° to 98.2°. If it falls below that even after her midcycle (postovulation), she may need thyroid for a while. Thyroid hormone helps open up the cell walls to let nutriments in, but the thyroid needs thyroid to help the thyroid make thyroid—a real catch-22. Kelp, because of its iodine content, might just do it; try five to ten tablets a day along with the foods high in B complex and see if things get moving again.

Q. I am seventeen and tend to gain easily. I have done the Weight Watchers thing, and it helps, but so slowly. Vitamins seem to increase my appetite. A lot of it is on my buttocks and thighs.

A. You may be one of those people who overproduces insulin when your blood sugar rises. The insulin pushes the blood sugar down, and you store the sugar as fat. The B vitamins will eventually help you burn up the fat. You might work on the theory that you are allergic to one of several foods—usually the ones you like. A food allergy can make the blood sugar bounce around just as much as eating naked sugar. Stop the milk and the beef, the two foods most likely to be interfering with your desired loss.

Q. I am a twenty-year-old female and have felt I was reasonably normal until about a year ago, when I began to have periods of depression lasting one to four days. There's no good reason; I just sit and bawl for hours. Pills help, but I hate the spacey feeling.

A. As I'm sure you know, counseling is the standard answer. You probably do need someone to guide you through all this and monitor your emotions. Diet is usually a factor if you have no pressing domestic or financial reasons for the symptoms. Hypoglycemia from sugar ingestion or from food allergy may explain it. Get someone to order a serum $B_{12}$ level. If it's low normal, a twice-weekly shot of $B_{12}$ should bring you out of your hole. Folic acid along with it might just make you perfect. Find a *holistic* doctor. If your depression is related to your menstrual periods extra $B_6$ might work better.

# Hyperactivity and Tension at All Ages  9

My work with hyperactive children led me to a new way of looking at all illnesses.

We were taught that these wild, restless, distractible children were the result of injuries to the nervous system at birth—cord about the neck, breech delivery, premature birth, collapsed lungs, and other toxic or anoxic insults. In time other parts of the nervous system would compensate for this damage.

It was discovered that most of these children could be calmed with stimulant drugs. Although this was only treating a symptom and not eliminating the cause, it was assumed that when obstetrics got "better" and the cause of premature birth was discovered, hyperactivity would disappear. It was also assumed that improving the poor academic performance of these children with drugs would prevent the development of the bad self-image that seemed to plague them throughout their lives.

About a decade ago I began to notice a gradual but

definite increase in the incidence of the hyperactive child. Teachers of my vintage told me that they were seeing five or six in every class in the late sixties where there had been only one or two per classroom in the late forties and early fifties. Was it the academic pressure on these children after Sputnik? Was it the crowded classrooms? Was it modern living? Was it a result of permissive child-rearing techniques? Or was it a diagnostic wastebasket for a variety of academic misfits? Any child who picked his nose in a class whose teacher had a low tolerance for nose-picking would be labeled hyperactive.

Did the teachers become more aware of hyperactivity because of their training and experience, or was it that the older teachers were becoming more intolerant of children just *breathing*? The increased incidence had to be some reflection of the "new" teaching pressures, because obstetrics was getting better. (The obstetricians claimed much less morbidity and mortality among the parturient.) Also, the new breed of neonatalists claimed increase of survival and decreased brain damage for premature infants.

So where were these wild and difficult-to-teach children coming from? The mothers of many of these obviously hyperactive children denied any delivery complications. Indeed, many of them indicated the child was acting up *before* delivery. (One father told me he was bruised by his hyperactive unborn child.)

Genetics had to be a factor, as was the quality of the pregnancy. This would help to explain the subtle and not-so-subtle differences in appearance and performance that make us unique individuals. Is there a gene for hyperactivity? Does it have to show up in every child of hyperactive parents? A child might appear normal to a family with a high activity level but be an obnoxious pest to a calm, quiet family. Rejection, indifference, or even hostility may be laid on these children because they do not fit into the family behavior pattern. A bad self-image, depression, or some form of sociopathy is frequently the end result for these unfortunate victims. (Seventy-five percent of prisoners in prisons today were hyperactive children according to a study done in 1974 by Maurice Bowerman.) Some effort must be applied early to discover and change these children since the benefits of psychotherapy on fixed patterns of thought and behavior are dubious at best.

Make the diagnosis before the diagnosis can be made. That sounds crazy, but it is really the basic tenet of preventive medicine. Students of alcoholism, antisocial behavior, reactive depression, suicide, and drug abuse all lay much etiological significance on early poor family, school, and peer relationships.

There are people more susceptible to certain illnesses than others. There is a genetic connection for most diseases and conditions. One out of four of us carries the gene for diabetes, but not all carriers come down with the full-blown disease. Some people who consume excess sodium (table salt) are very likely to get high blood pressure, so we tell everybody to go easy on salt intake, especially those in families who have a history of high blood pressure, strokes, and other vascular trouble.

In our "search for truth," then, we must be vigilant and detect the children with early signs of the problem but also know what environmental and genetic factors might make some children more susceptible than others. Not that hyperactivity is *bad*, but in the wrong situations it becomes a negative factor in child rearing. An inherent danger in any prognostic proclamation laid on a child is that the child tends to fulfill the prophecy. This tendency to become the label is real, and I don't want to catch any blame for being a party to its fulfillment. Just say it's possible to be hyper and get a bad self-image, but it may be neat to be the proud parents of an Edison, an Einstein, or a Winston Churchill.

The bottom line in rearing any child is to give him a good self-image.

Somehow the child has to believe (feel, perceive, realize, be overwhelmingly assured) that he is a decent (worthwhile, wanted, will-be-cared-for, nice-to-have-around) human being. Someone has to tell him this. Words are a help, but actions are more meaningful. Rocking, caressing, feeding, changing, smiling at, laughing with, imitating the sounds of, bathing, rubbing, massaging, and burping are but a few of the early things we parents must do and must enjoy doing or the child will perceive or suspect he is persona non grata, an unwanted guest.

There are a number of things hyper children do that may get in the way of enthusiastic acceptance by their parents. And if the parents—who may have headaches, depression, or quick tempers also—are having trouble with their own minds and bodies, they may find it difficult to continue to reward the child for his presence, much less his actions. (I love the way you wake up every morning at two o'clock.)

My experience with all children, but especially those with hyperactive tendencies, has given me the opportunity to correlate early childhood traits with adult symptoms. Many "behavior problems" in children are now known to be caused by biochemical or nutritional imbalances that, if not solved at the metabolic level at an early age, may become psychiatric problems requiring lengthy and costly therapy that is frequently no better than handholding because it ignores chemical facts of life. (If you are weak because of anemia, a friendly psychotherapeutic session may make you feel better about it and even digest your food better, but the first order of business is to eat foods containing iron and then find out why you became anemic in the first place.)

The following observable conditions are clues that a nutritional approach would be helpful. Ticklish, sensitive children cannot keep the environment at a safe distance. Excess stimuli come into the perceiving part of the brain's cortex, and messages are sent to the body to alert the glands and muscles that something extraordinary is going on out there.

If these end organs are overly used, especially the adrenals which respond to stress, they can become exhausted, and symptoms will develop that vary with the exhausted organ. Organ susceptibility to stress is determined by genetic factors, but it can be assuaged if the end organs are refreshed with appropriate nutrients.

Instead of just treating the asthma, the migraine, the arthritis, the rash, some effort should be devoted toward eliminating the stress, making the filtering mechanism more efficient, helping the cortex become less sensitive, and providing amino acids, vitamins, minerals, oxygen, and fuel to the weakened tissues.

Hyperactive children are unable to ignore unimportant stimuli. These children are upset by minor changes. The birth process is a major traumatic shock, even though everyone was as gentle as possible. He acts as if he were plunged into ice water when he perceives the change of temperature on his skin. His mother tries to cuddle and comfort him, and he screams inconsolably; he is sure he is going to die. Then he notices his mother's breasts coming, and he may think he will suffocate. In his paranoia he may stiff-arm the very people who are trying to love and comfort him. Many mothers will "get the message" and give up by backing off and propping a bottle or feeding at arm's length because that is what the baby is telling the world: "You are too close." Of course, these are the very children who should be breast-fed because the same biochemical fault that allows them to be so goosey is related to the biochemical mechanism behind much of the allergic state and susceptibility to infection.

Colic to them is an appendicitis attack. A bit of

postnasal drip makes them vomit. They sneeze six times instead of two. When tipped up for a diaper change, they are panicked as if in an earthquake. Cutting teeth allows them to get bronchitis. They are exquisitely sensitive to food, air, and bath temperature. They usually hate being cuddled. They appear to be suspicious. If stimulated, rocked, massaged, or tickled, they may respond with uncontrolled laughter, shrieking until they throw up. The family learns to use a controlled approach. Vomiting may be a body language that says "You are getting close again!"

The family learns by this behavior-modification mechanism that they have a touchy child. If you toss your child lovingly into the air a few times in the evening and the child cannot sleep all night, you have learned not to throw your child into the air. The child may perceive this backing off by his caretakers and assume it is rejection.

Babies delivered by something close to the Le Boyer (quiet) birth process, who were allowed to nurse immediately, received no solids for the first eight to twelve months, and had close and constant contact with both parents, seem to be more secure and have fewer allergies and infections than those who were delivered traumatically, did not receive the early attachment, and were bottle-fed.

These observations by medical and La Leche League leaders may not prove that nursing is ideal for humans (it does make sense); it may only indicate that some babies are amenable to nursing because of genetic, pregnancy, and delivery factors. The baby's and mother's nursing abilities reinforce the cuddling and pleasurable aspects of the closeness.

Some long-term observations must be made to see if the babies who need distance and are telling us to step back a pace, who resist and resent the rules of home and school, will always grow up to be troublemakers, mavericks, or restless loners whose theme song is "Is That All There Is?"

We are social animals, and although being alone and

doing one's thing is rewarding, we *do* need others for love, praise, and communication, to see where we are occasionally. Social interaction should be fun, a joy. If a baby cries a lot from gas and anxiety and his parents hold him because they feel sorry for him and want to help because they love this helpless creature, is it possible that the baby may perceive the parents as the *source* of his distress? The parents may think they are cuddling him because he is crying. The baby may associate crying with cuddling and may learn it is better to fight out his problem alone.

In the last ten years, since I have been paying particular attention to these touchy children, I have only found two or three children from a group of about five thousand hyperactives who were *not* ticklish. On a scale of 1 to 4+, these restless children who cannot sit still in school, who are disruptive and frequently discipline problems, are 3 to 4+ ticklish. Not every ticklish child is hyperactive, but from the ranks of the ticklish ones come the children who are unable to disregard unimportant stimuli.

During my examination the light bothers their eardrums; just to look at the tongue blade makes them gag; feeling for swollen glands in the neck or throat is stimulating; and, of course, the warm stethoscope is cold. They are so ticklish that my soft warm hand on their abdomen makes them double up with laughter and occasionally fall off the examining table.

When I discover this phenomenon, I turn to the mother (usually) and ask "Trouble in school?"

"Trouble in school," is the affirmation.

The hernia check is usually out of the question.

During the history-taking and the question-and-answer period I note in almost all these children some past clue, some symptom, some sign predictive of their present educational dysfunction.

Colicky, fussy, sensitive, wakeful, restless, whined a

lot, rocked, sucked, never relaxed, touched everything, gregarious, never satisfied, uncuddleable, crabby, stubborn, pouty, talkative, easily stimulated by crowds, noises, sights, walked without crawling are but a few of the things parents can observe that *may* be harbingers of later social and educational maladjustments.

If the child has been brought to me because of unsatisfactory school performance and is accompanied by a note from the teacher, the situation has come to a crisis. Something must be done. The teacher has exhausted all her or his educational tricks in attempting to motivate the child to sit still and learn. The school wants him on a pill or referred to a psychiatrist.

We were trained in medical school to place these children on a medicine known as Ritalin®, Dexedrine® or Cylert®, and if it had a calming effect and stretched out his attention span, then the rest was up to the school. The drug made him school-ready. If he still was uneducable, then he had dyslexia, was retarded, or had a psychiatric block.

This was all predicated on the supposition that the children so afflicted had been hurt at birth. The drug would hold them together until some other part of the nervous system matured sufficiently to compensate for the deficiency. No one knew why the stimulant had a calming effect. As a matter of fact, this paradoxical sedating effect with the use of stimulants was discovered by error.

Some feel that the stimulant facilitates or stimulates some learning or attention center in the cerebral cortex. Some evidence from animal studies indicates that it enhances or prolongs the effect of a natural brain chemical, norepinephrine, a stimulant found predominantly in an area of the lower brain (limbic system) concerned with filtering out extraneous stimuli so that every stimulus does not *have* to arrive at the cortex.

It seems that genetic factors and pregnancy insults as

well as obstetrical complications can all lead singly or in combination to the same set of symptoms: a touchy child with a short attention span who is unable to disregard unimportant stimuli.

The fact that at least five times as many boys as girls are hyperactive suggests genetic factors are operative, since the birth process cannot selectively injure boys more than girls. However, this 5-to-1 ratio may be spurious because a hyperactive girl may be more orally hyper while the boy is more likely to be motor-driven and have to use his legs, which would make him more noticeable and therefore counted.

I find in my series of cases that blue-eyed blonds, green-eyed redheads, and hazel-eyed fair children outnumber the brown-eyed brunets, Jews, and Orientals by a factor of three to one. Of the brown-eyed hyper children, half are of American Indian extraction, and the other half did have some fairly obvious nervous-system hurt at birth or shortly thereafter. Not all blue-eyed children are ticklish and not all Indians are hyper, and some fair children did have obvious noxious episodes that might have allowed the syndrome to develop.

We now have enough information—folk, scientific, and anecdotal—to be able to assign some nutritional and biochemical deficiencies to many physical symptoms and disturbing behaviors before some overt disease becomes manifest.

Some years ago a doctor in Idaho told me he was treating hyperactive children with thyroid hormone. I could understand the use of a stimulant to calm these restless ones, but I had never realized that low thyroid production could be a feature of the hyperactive syndrome. He said many such children test out at the low end of the normal range for thyroid function. I checked a few of my patients but found nothing consistent or reliable. A blind alley.

But now I wonder if he wasn't on to something. These children eat vast amounts of food but yet stay thin; if a normal person ate that much, he would gain a pound an hour. We know that the thyroid hormone has a regulating effect on every cell of the body, and one function of this ubiquitous chemical is to "open up the cell walls" and let the nutrients in.

Dr. Broda Barnes has shown us how common hypofunction of the thyroid is. Perhaps low body temperature in the morning plus voracious appetite plus a thin body build plus hyperactivity might be put together as an equation that means hypothyroidism. The slow heart rate and constipation of so many of these children would tend to substantiate the diagnosis. The laboratory is not perfect.

Many patients suffering from hypothyroid function have low levels of the various minerals in their hair. Patients complaining of needing vast amounts of sleep and still having fatigue are more likely to be low in iron, copper, manganese, zinc, and chromium, the minerals that help trigger in the body enzymes involved in energy production. Although they eat a lot, they are not *absorbing* the foods well. Some patients improve overnight by taking pancreatic digestive enzymes with each meal.

We started to do hair tests on some hyperactive children because it was reported that two of the signs of lead poisoning were hyperactivity and educational dysfunction. This phenomenon is found in inner cities, some ghetto areas, and along heavily traveled freeways, presumably from the exhaust of lead-containing fuel, the burning of lead storage batteries, and leaching of lead from water pipes. We are seeing a fairly high relationship between hyperactivity, low calcium, and low magnesium in the hair, a high incidence of rhythmical habits, plus a craving for dairy products. As a matter of fact, the more the craving, the more likely the child's hair test to be low in calcium. It is as if they know where the calcium is and consume it, but apparently cannot absorb it.

So many hyper children seemed to crave milk and dairy products almost as much as sugar, and so many of their hair tests seemed to be low in calcium that there appeared to be a relationship. The hyper ones who had some rhythmical tension-relieving activity were more likely to be low in calcium and have this craving for milk. These are the thumb-suckers, the bed-rockers, the hair-twisters, the ear-lobe-pullers, the nail-biters, the navel-pickers, the foot-swingers and leg-bouncers.

We were taught in medical school that these were insecure children because if you pulled the thumb or pacifier out of their mouths, they would cry. They had to do their rhythmical thing. A fresh idea has come along that I like; it is called the Gate Theory. We have sensory impulses coming into our cortex from our eyes, ears, nose, mouth, body, muscles, and if these are too many or too strong, they tend to change our brain waves from alpha (comfortable) to beta (uncomfortable). Most of us have found ways to stay on alpha waves (booze, smoking, meditation, prayer, hot baths, eating, jogging, and so on), but children have to make do with what they have: rocking the bed or sucking the thumb. The message from the back, the knees, the thumb, gums, or lips up to the brain says "You're OK, you're OK," and this shuts the gate on the other, presumably irritating messages from the world or the gassy intestines: "You're not OK; you're not OK!"

The limbic system, which is supposed to filter out unimportant stimuli, is probably basically at fault because it allows too many stimuli in to crowd the cortex. When the cortex gets too many messages, it assumes some stress is at work and so alerts the pituitary, which in turn sets the whole body up for flight or fight. So the rhythmical motor activity is a stress-saver.

I wonder also if a part of the story could be explained this way: Since many of these children appear to be low in calcium, and since spastic, twitching muscles are due to very low calcium (tetany), maybe these rocking, sucking, biting, banging children are telling us they have tight, sensitive muscles. Some, indeed, have painful shin splints, muscle cramps, and tight-neck and back spasms. If they are taken to the doctor with these complaints, they get aspirin, bed rest, and a diagnosis of "growing pains." Or worse: "He's trying to get out of something." It is amazing how rapidly and easily and cheaply these complaints respond to calcium and sometimes magnesium. Most of these low-calcium victims who crave milk give histories suggesting a lifelong milk-allergy problem—colic, vomiting, eczema, plugged nose, cough, asthma, bronchitis, ear infections, constipation, diarrhea, hives, bedwetting, strep throats, croup, cracks about the anus. I am assuming that it all means that the victim is still allergic to milk and the intestines cannot absorb the calcium from cow's milk but can from calcium lactate, bone meal, or goat's milk. I have many patients who have no trouble from raw, certified milk, but their symptoms recur if they drink homogenized, pasteurized cow's milk. Someone is doing something to the milk that wrecks it for some people.

A twenty-eight-year-old I know had complained all her life about aches and pains but had been told to "stop faking it!" She was miserable every day until she hurt her shoulder on the job two years ago and was given Empirin with codeine as a temporary painkiller while her torn muscles healed.

Within one hour of that first pill she was hooked— "I've never felt this good in my whole life!" When the prescription was used up she enthusiastically announced to her doctor what a terrific diagnostician and therapist he was—and "Please, may I have some more?"

"Of course not. Your shoulder is healed, so there should be no more pain. And codeine is a narcotic. I can't just pass out drugs like that." She worked out a little exchange of services with him and for two years she took ten to fifteen pills a day. She felt awful when she took them and awful without them.

I gave her a few vitamin C, B complex, and calcium injections intravenously over a four-week period, and she was able to get off her dope with few withdrawal side effects. She still remembers how good that first pill was and even tried the codeine again. She is happy and comfortable with her body now but remembers with bitterness the putdowns by parents, siblings, and doctors.

There is no way we are able to live inside someone else's body. We must accept this restriction and use whatever clues are available. All her life she had been trying to tell her mother, her teacher, and her doctor that she was low in calcium, at least, the B vitamins, and—of course—vitamin C. She sucked her thumb a lot as an infant. She rocked. She craved milk most of her life. She had many ear infections from one to five years of age. These are usually the clues about milk allergy. She had her tonsils and adenoids removed because of the repeated sore throats. The surgery is a stress, and stress depletes the adrenals and calcium is lost. She had many aches and pains and frequently awakened with a stiff neck. She felt nervous and despondent, and had insomnia from age twelve to sixteen years. She tried such drugs as speed, marijuana, and LSD, but they did not keep pain away. She was often bedridden during her periods because of the severity of the cramping.

I used to use cod-liver oil tablets (five per day for a week) when parents reported muscle cramps and growing pains. It helped because it improved calcium absorption. How many older people are complaining of aches and pains and are bent forward because of low calcium? And they are afraid the calcium will make their joints stiff! We all need calcium and magnesium until the day we die (well, maybe until two or three days before we go).

## Questions and Answers

**Q. What is a hyperactive child?**

**A.** This is a child who is unable to disregard unimportant stimuli to the point that he is put down, ignored, and punished by parents, teachers, and peer group. (The condition is now called Attention Deficit Disorder.) If he has nothing that makes him feel decent and worthwhile (hobby, sports, music) and he is hearing commands ("Don't do that," "Sit down," "Go to bed") and questions ("What did you do that for?" "Where are you going now?") twice as often as he is getting compliments or mere acceptance, he is in danger of developing a poor self-image that could plague him and distort his relations with others for the rest of his life.

**Q. Are there different grades of hyperactivity?**

**A.** Yes. They range on a continuum from normal alertness and saying "Ouch!" when stuck with a pin to the child who cannot read because the child sitting next to him is breathing. Some children are comfortable at home and have a normal attention span but fall apart at school because thirty children in the class quietly sitting there is something he cannot ignore. If a child has more trouble at home with his parents, it is not classic hyperactivity; it may be an emotional problem. He is supposed to have more problems when or where the distractions are more numerous.

**Q. What happens to hyper kids?**

**A.** Most of them grow up and become ordinary citizens, a little restless, and in general they find it difficult to nest. The ones who survive and achieve the best are those who somehow developed a good self-image, who are fairly cheerful (sometimes the class clown), and who do not have too much trouble reading. Dr. Charles L. Shedd noticed a relationship between criminality and nonreading. He felt that the conscience and the reading center are close to each other in the neocortex. It appears that depressed, grumpy nonreaders are more likely to end up as criminals with depressions.

I find many happy and successful people in rewarding jobs and professions who freely admit to having been hyper in school. Radio and televison talk-show hosts were usually hyper kids. Flight attendants, truck drivers, and people who end up in "moving" jobs were in general restless kids. And so, probably, was Attila the Hun. Most hyper kids tend to avoid higher education because of the long, boring study and class hours. Maybe this is why doctors tend to be unsympathetic; they are relatively free of the problem or they would not have gone on so long with higher education (although I know a hyper surgeon who prided himself on an eighteen-minute appendectomy).

Q. Can hyper adults be treated?

A. They may never outgrow the genetic love of motion and the strong need to win and the never-satisfied feelings, but they can live more comfortably if they watch their diets. Hyper adults can be treated, although preferably not with drugs. If the bad self-image is present, psychotherapy may be needed. But the restless legs, the allergies, the insomnia, the highs and lows to which hyper people are susceptible can usually be controlled with nutrition.

Q. If a child does well academically but has behavior problems, is he hyper?

A. Many hyper children can do well in school because they read well and are bright, but they *are* a disturbance. Schools should make an effort to give them extra projects or have them spend time in the library. If forced to sit still in class, the child will get bored and disruptive. Then the teacher has to discipline him, and he learns to hate school.

It is true that behavior problems are more likely to be seen in hyperactive children because they respond to stress in a motoric way. Schools must compromise with these children who need to move more than their class-mates; the feeling of self-worth is more important than the academic education.

**Q. If a child is not hyper, will he become so if he eats the wrong food?**

**A.** Not necessarily. Lots of kids eat sugar and white-flour products and appear to function satisfactorily. (Some-day they will acquire their family problem, arthritis, obe-sity, allergies, or diabetes, because their organs cannot cope after a period of malnutrition.) Some are temporarily hyper after Easter and Halloween because of the carbohydrate load then but are just ordinary kids the rest of the year. The ones who seem to have the trouble are the genetically tainted, the neurologically hurt, and the ones with low calcium. They are all ready to become hyper, then the carbohydrate diet or the ingestion of an allergen sets off the pancreas' overresponse.

**Q. When should parents tell the school their child is hyper?**

**A.** In general, it is best to let the teacher figure it out for himself or herself. If a child is labeled—especially if the teacher has a low threshold for hyperactivity—the child becomes the label and is sunk for the whole year. Some teachers love the challenge of working with the "difficult" students. The principal may be helpful: he or she can place the child in a more appropriate classroom. One of my patients needed three Dexedrine® tablets for one teacher and none for the next.

**Q. How does the problem show itself in different age groups?**

**A.** The global statement about these children is that they are unable to disregard unimportant stimuli; therefore they notice sights, sounds, temperature changes, tactile stimuli, muscle, intestine, bladder, and perhaps bone sensations more than other children of the same age. Hospital nursery nurses know; mothers of two or three children know even before birth. Two mothers swear that during their pregnancies their unborn hyper children kicked them out of bed. Maybe having your child stay all day with a mother of four or five and getting her diagnosis will help. The supermarket clerk can spot them. The doctor usually cannot tell. The point seems to be that if the child is getting on your nerves and you are unable to say something nice twice as often as you put him down, you need help. If this book does not get you both straightened out, then professional help is required.

**Q. If a child is hyper because of "brain damage" from a difficult delivery, will diet and vitamins control it?**

**A.** A nutritional program will help, but if the problem is severe, special educational facilities and medication will be necessary. Almost everybody can be made to function better. Since vitamins and minerals help enzymes and enzymes do the work of the body, it makes sense to try the nutritional support system first. If a stimulant helps calm a child, then I assume the enzyme that produces norepinephrine is not operating optimally, and nutrition usually will help it produce the required amounts.

**Q. Can you use prescribed drugs along with nutrition?**

**A.** Many parents find they *have* to. Some children have such a problem that the combined effects of a special class, enough stimulants to wreck the appetite, and a vitamin B complex shot every day makes them barely tolerable. At the same time the child is supposed to be getting the message that all this effort is for him and that he is worthwhile.

Many parents of my patients know that diet is an answer but, because they feel it is too difficult to maintain due to their own or their spouse's or children's cravings for sugar, have found it easier to give the kid a pill than fight to get a wholesome breakfast down.

Some have found that the nutritional program is quite satisfactory and the whole family is better (less sick and more cheerful), but there are "days." Some find prescribed pills are necessary on stress or test days. It's supposed to be cheating to take it before an athletic performance. In general, however, these medications act as downers and might impede performance.

**Q. Are many adopted children hyperactive?**

**A.** Many are. Ten percent of hyper children are adopted while only 1 percent of the population is adopted. (About 15 to 20 percent of the child population are hyper.) The reasons may be varied. Genetic factors may prevent the biological parents from desiring to nest. The pregnant woman may not have eaten properly for a variety of reasons. Age and physical and mental stress could have taken their toll. Prenatal care may not have been optimum. Many adoptive parents feel guilty that the child is so unmanageable and often assume it is because they are not the biological parents. I see more allergies in adopted children, perhaps from stress and poor diet in the pregnancy but also because many adopting mothers are unwilling to nurse the adoptee.

**Q. Can a hyper mother make her child hyper by example?**

**A.** Usually if it is not the child's basic personality, hyper by example doesn't happen. A prominent hyper television performer told me she used to awaken her daughter at 2 A.M. to get her to take an extra milkshake because she did not think the child was eating enough during the day. It did not affect the girl; as a matter of fact, she learned to turn her mother off with quiet, stoical, nonresponse self-control. Most children learn to cope in their own way with domestic decibels, but if they do not have a good nervous-system screening device, it will affect them.

**Q. How do I get my doctor to examine for hyperactivity or do something about it? My child's teacher says he is hyper; my doctor says no medicine.**

A. Hyperactivity is only in the observer's eye; he didn't see it because he doesn't go to school with your child. A note from the teacher may help him change his mind, but he may then only offer some drug. That's OK and may be a help in establishing the diagnosis. If the medicine works, assume that some brain enzyme is not working well and the child needs a diet change and extra B complex and calcium. Use the medicine if it works to allow the child and the teacher to make some progress and have some success. The nutritional approach takes about three weeks, so you should be able to taper off on the drug during that time and maybe eventually not use any at all. It is best not to use it on weekends unless they are stressful. Most patients are able to reduce the dose of medicine 70 to 100 percent in the three weeks it takes the nutritional approach to work. The doctors who will believe you are the ones that have hyper kids themselves. At least find a supportive doctor.

**Q. Can bad eyes cause hyperactivity?**

A. No doubt about it. Double vision, nearsightedness, and farsightedness, if associated with dysperception, will lead to discouragement. But many kids with bad eyes are not hyper. Some children cannot explain to us that the letters are not clear; the letter *a* may fill up his whole visual angle, and we are asking him to pronounce the whole word *and*. Some optometrists may be helpful. It is important to figure out if the child's visual skills come and go; if so, diet and fluctuating blood sugar levels must be attended to first.

If the child can see but cannot read because he cannot remember the sounds of the letters, his memory may be at fault. Ask if he can remember his dreams. If not, add B$_6$ (50 to 200 mg per day) to his improved diet. In a couple of days he should be catching on.

Many reading specialists can give an accurate diagnostic profile. You may find the local chapter of the Association for Children with Learning Disabilities very helpful. Usually the hyperactivity prevents the child from learning to read. Hearing defects, even a few minor ear infections at critical times in a child's development, can lead to learning disabilities.

**Q. My pediatrician diagnosed hyperactivity in my sixteen-month-old. Isn't that rather early? He did stop napping at one year. At what age can an accurate diagnosis be made?**

A. The diagnosis is one of observation. It often is a general "feeling" that this child right here in this room is more restless than the last twelve who came through. Pediatricians see a stream of children every day, twenty to thirty, in all sizes and degrees of panic, hope, fear, courage, stoicism. One does get impressions after a few years of the parade. The doctor may be right. The ticklish, overly sensitive ones are more likely to have the trouble, but one cannot decide until school and the stress of sitting still are forced on the child. Then decide. Doctors like to play the predictive game.

In any case—but clearly depending on your relationship with the child—it would be worthwhile, and hence the reason for this book, to do a few things now and see if the child is calmer at the next checkup with the doctor. Maybe just stopping the milk and sugar and adding some calcium at nap- and bedtime will be sufficient for the borderline case. But maybe the *doctor* is the stress.

**Q. How do you discipline a hyperactive child? Is it different from disciplining a normal child?**

A. All children need discipline, but some of these

wild ones only get punishment. Indeed, the hyper child in the family is more likely to be the battered one. It is hard to get upset with a child who breaks some clearly established rule and then smiles winsomely and says "Gee, I'm sorry." Most authorities agree that some immediate and appropriate action should be taken for transgressions. But first try to find out what part of the nervous system you are dealing with, the cortex where social rules are stored or the limbic system where there is no conscience. Maybe your child threw the garbage on the floor because you asked him to take the garbage out when his blood sugar had dipped and you were asking a gorilla to do the job. A quick dollop of protein and twenty minutes of "time out" (like hockey players need occasionally) should restore your child (or spouse) to his usual pleasant, cortex-in-charge self. If you cannot blame diet, maybe the child just doesn't feel well (infection, worms, anemia, odd brain waves).

Q. I have a blue-eyed, blond, ticklish son whose father's family is full of diabetes, obesity, and alcoholism. Will hyper symptoms show up before age four years?

A. They don't have to show up at all. Maybe he's hyper and you don't know it because your husband is and you can tolerate these restless people. His first-grade teacher may have another way of looking at children and may not like gregarious, active children. Your son may be OK until he gets hit with an allergy or he is stressed with excess carbohydrates.

Q. My seven-year-old still has bowel movements in his underwear. He is a little hyper, has few friends, claims he doesn't know when he does it. It is disgusting and embarrassing. Getting mad does not help. Making him wash his own things makes no difference.

A. This is called encopresis (which is Greek for soiling oneself and looks better in medical journals). The psychiatrists say it is a form of passive aggression. The child feels put upon by the world and is paying it back. The treatment is to teach the child to be orally assertive so he won't be anally aggressive. Sometimes it works. Some of us have had good results with a nutrition approach. Assume that his cortex is not getting the message that his rectum is ready to empty because of so many other incoming stimuli, plus low blood sugar from poor diet or ingestion of allergens. Assume also that milk is sludging him up so he gets confusing messages from his colon. Stop all dairy products. No rice, potatoes, or low-roughage foods. Make him sit on the toilet for at least fifteen to twenty minutes after breakfast and really try. Let him get verbally hostile also; it could help. Extra B vitamins, calcium, and maybe a touch of Milk of Magnesia® may help his cortex—where the message is stored: "Don't poop in your pants; mother doesn't like it."

**Q. I'm a teacher. I see these kids all the time. I know they are bright and could learn easily if they would sit still for three minutes. I see the result of candy ingestion— birthdays and after Easter and Halloween. How can I get the parents to change the diet without upsetting them or making them think they are bad parents?**

**A.** That's a tough question, because you are getting no support from the child's doctor that there is a connection between candy and hyperactivity. Most teacher-parent conferences are supposed to air these possibilities, but give the good news first. "We love Charlie; he dresses well, contributes a lot to the class, has friends, does well in sports, but. . . ." And be sure the bad news equals the good news. "He could do so much better if he would sit still. He has good and bad days, he is behind in his multiplication tables, and some days he seems out of touch. Does he like sweets and junk food? Some other children have been that way and when their diet was changed" (don't say "were given a better diet") "they improved. Could he be allergic to something?" Smile a lot!

My job is to keep talking to people until everyone understands that diet has a lot to do with the way we feel and act. Maybe a lesson plan that would involve the children would help. For instance, have your class come one day with no breakfast, let everyone eat sixteen marshmallows and then be their own observers. The next day they would have protein or vegetables and then compare performance with the preceding day. Children often believe the teacher faster than they believe their parents.

**Q. We love our five-year-old, but he cannot give up his thumb-sucking and hair-twisting. We are embarrassed because he appears shy and insecure when he does this, especially if tired, bored, or in a strange place. I know my mother-in-law thinks I'm not quite the perfect person to take care of her grandson. He doesn't do this when he is with her. We've ignored it, scolded him, put dye on to remind him, and had our dentist talk to him. It works for five minutes.**

**A.** I'm amazed at how many children do these irritating rhythmical things and grow up to be perfectly normal adults. My feeling is that as we grow we substitute other calming activities as a replacement for something as childish as sucking or rocking. We still need the patterned movement but we use "adult" actions: smoking, combing, grooming, tapping fingers, cracking knuckles, swinging a leg, jiggling a foot up and down, disco dancing, chewing gum, and talking.

These activities must be blocking out uncomfortable incoming stimuli that the cortex cannot handle. Assume that he cannot screen out stimuli. Change his diet, stop milk if he loves it, and add calcium, magnesium, and a good supply of B complex vitamins; they all help make the brain chemicals that run his filtering system.

**Q. Our four-year-old daughter rocks the bed with a pillow between her legs. She will go faster and faster, then**

gets all hot, stares into space, and relaxes and goes to sleep. It looks sexy. Isn't she too young for that?

A. Not at all. It's called self-stimulation, autoeroticism, or masturbation. It is considered a normal developmental phenomenon and prepares the individual for adult sexual activities—sort of "practice makes perfect." Try not to show any sense of disgust or shame.

If children prefer the activity to normal social play, a problem is present. Usually, however, some irritation draws their attention to the area: a bladder infection, a food allergy, pinworms, a contact rash from bubble-bath soap, dry skin. Orange juice, chocolate, and milk are the most common foods that set up the itch. When the child scratches the itch, other pleasant pathways are stimulated.

Try the foods that control allergies; that includes calcium. See if the self-stimulation is less necessary. (Could milk be an aphrodisiac?)

Q. My eleven-month-old baby is breast-fed except for a night bottle. She sucks her thumb so vigorously and constantly that I can hardly get the solid food into her. She doesn't particularly care for solids, but I worry about milk anemia. I used to think it was terrible that people let their babies suck on things. Now I've got one who's an expert. How do you get them to stop?

A. We've tried to get people to get babies used to a pacifier that fits the contour of the upper gum. It pushes the teeth around less than the bony thumb, and it is something that can be discarded by the child on his own timetable.

She may be telling you that you are being too pushy about solids (and other things). Back off and just have fun with her. Don't be so serious or she will think she is not completely acceptable. She is old enough for table food; she may want to feed herself.

Try calcium anyway. Maybe the milk and the solids

are giving her a stomachache and sucking is her tranquilizer. Breast milk usually has enough iron for babies.

There is a rule: The more you pay attention to some disagreeable habit, the more your child will perpetuate it.

**Q. I know my fourteen-year-old boy is trying out cigarettes, pot, alcohol, and drugs. He has not been the perfect student. Teachers would say "I know he could do better if he would try." He is looking for acceptance from his peers who all seem to be headed into the hands of the devil. Counselors say "Give him freedom within the rules." The police can do nothing until he speeds or wrecks property or steals. My minister has tried. My doctor says "A phase." I'm afraid he'll get hooked on the big H. Do I have to just watch him destroy himself?**

A. We are all to blame for these youngsters who slip away from our influence. We treat them like children but expect them to be grown up. Their bodies are growing rapidly, and we allow them to eat vitaminless and mineral-depleted calories. They don't feel good. School is a drag. The parents know that if they would eat better they would feel better, but the adolescent hates to admit his parents are right.

Most junior high and high school students try illicit drugs because of peer pressure and curiosity. If they feel better on the drug, it is no wonder they continue it. The hypoglycemic, tired, depressed ones will find alcohol may be perfect. The hyper kid may shoot speed and get calmed. The low-calcium, restless one will find narcotics are his answer.

We must feed them better, and we must axe the candy and pop machines in the schools. We cannot let them decide what to eat; they are too hungry to choose anything but quick carbohydrates. There is a federal regulation now to help: no candy sold until the lunch is served. Call your school and find out if it is being enforced.

But what to do about your son? He needs a counselor, a nutritionist, a change of school, or a sabbatical work year, some understanding and prayer. He needs to win— somehow, somewhere.

## Recipes with Calcium, Magnesium, and B Complex Vitamins

Calcium deficiency is reasonably common in our country. Dairy products are the traditional vehicle for the ingestion of the 1000 mg a day each human should have. Many other foods are full of calcium, but many children dislike them.

Calcium and magnesium combine with oxalic acid to make oxalates, which make the calcium and magnesium largely unavailable for absorption and use by the body. If one is trying to increase the amounts of these minerals, avoid beet greens, spinach, Swiss chard, and rhubarb as the oxalates will bind the calcium in them and the minerals will pass on through the intestines. The oxalates in tea, coffee, and chocolate when consumed with calcium and magnesium will prevent the absorption of some of the calcium and magnesium. Chocolate milk is illogical in its concept and dangerous in its ingestion. The extent to which oxalates and phytates bind with calcium and magnesium in other foods (i.e. nuts, legumes, and cereal grains) is probably not sufficient to have a significant effect.

Sesame seeds contain ten times per weight the amount of calcium in milk, but the unhulled seeds must be used because most of the calcium is in the hull. For those with a milk allergy, a pound of these seeds can be blended and made into four quarts of Sesame Milk (page 119). Use this as a milk substitute in recipes such as shakes and frozen popsicles. The price is equal to or below that of milk, and the calcium content is much higher.

Sesame Butter (page 128) is called tahini; it is

somewhat strong in taste but is much more creamy than natural peanut butter. Try combining ½ cup natural peanut butter with ½ cup sesame butter and 1 or 2 tablespoons of honey. The resulting mixture will be creamier than the plain peanut butter and loaded with calcium.

Other great sources of calcium are Parmesan, Swiss, and brick cheeses. Children with milk allergies can often tolerate cheese. If your child is *able* to eat cheese, serve him foods with a high potassium content along with his meal or snack containing cheese. (Some good sources of potassium are raisins, bananas, dried apricots, figs, peaches, and raw sunflower seeds.) The reason for this is that the cheeses contain a large amount of sodium, which needs to be counteracted by a proportionately larger amount of potassium for the balance.

Other foods with good amounts of calcium: dry whey powder, torula yeast, dry carob powder, dry soy milk, raw parsley, low-fat soy grits, raw almonds, dried figs, dry raw soybeans, brewer's yeast, raw hazelnuts, garbanzos (chickpeas).

Be sure to drain cooked spinach and greens thoroughly so that the oxalic acid they contain will be drained off as much as possible.

Because yogurt is made from milk (goat's milk or reconstituted dry milk is best) that has been scalded to destroy all bacteria before the yogurt culture is added, it is often tolerated by milk-intolerant children. Its calcium content will fortify any milk-containing recipe. Invest in a yogurt-maker if your child can eat yogurt. A quick, nutritious breakfast kids love is a bowl of plain yogurt with fruit, nuts, or seeds, granola and dried fruit, or all of these. Let them create their own "sundaes" and they'll gobble down their breakfast.

Dolomite (limestone) also fortifies recipes with calcium, but care must be taken to hide it in foods with a stronger taste and texture, such as peanut butter.* Another clever way to add calcium to the diet is to follow the recipe for soup stock, then add it to stews, gravies, and the water for cooking vegetables. Be sure to add the vinegar—it draws the calcium out of the bones. Make up a pot and freeze it in ice trays for easy accessibility.

Calcium and magnesium work together in the body. Foods that provide the best source of magnesium include dry raw wheat germ and bran, natural raw almonds, cashew nuts, dry raw soy beans, soy milk, low-fat soy grits, brewer's yeast, raw buckwheat, raw Brazil nuts, raw peanuts, raw hazelnuts, raw whole sesame seeds, lima beans, whole-grain millet, rolled oats, pecans, walnuts, and lentils.

Herbs that provide both calcium and magnesium would include blue cohosh, cayenne, dandelion, and red raspberry leaves. Kelp and alfalfa are also sources.

A teaspoon of dolomite has about the same amount of calcium as does a quart of milk. Dolomite has magnesium and bone meal does not. Lactose helps calcium absorption. A high-protein diet cuts down on calcium absorption, and calcium will also be lost in the urine. Calcium is lost if stress is high and exercise is low. Fat in the diet cuts down on calcium absorption.

Even with a good source of calcium, only about 40 percent of that ingested is absorbed. (More than 80 percent of fractures occur in postmenopausal women; the chronic calcium loss over the years allows this susceptibility.)

If we could just get everyone to eat some liver once a week, we would all be better. Along with vitamin A, it has big amounts of the B complex. The B complex vitamins are helpful for those with fatigue or who are under stress or have memory trouble. Almost every physical and mental symptom has been ascribed to low B complex intake.

* Beware of possible contaminant trace metals in dolomite compounds.

Brewer's yeast, or nutritional yeast as it is often called, contains an equally impressive amount of B vitamins, and recipes can easily be fortified by it. Use brewer's yeast in dishes with lots of liquid, since it tends to absorb liquids. The taste is strong but not unpalatable. Add a little at a time, tasting as you go along to insure that its flavor does not overpower the taste of the dish in question.

B complex is also found abundantly in wheat germ (buy the kind grown on blackstrap molasses; it tastes the best by far) and bran, green vegetables, peanuts, egg yolks, and whole grains. In addition, pantothenic acid ($B_5$) can be found in peas, beans, and raw mushrooms, while pyridoxine ($B_6$) is contained in bananas, avocados, rice polishings, walnuts, cantaloupe, cabbage, peppers, carrots, and pecans. Pyridoxine is destroyed by cooking, so if you are attempting to fortify your supply, be sure to eat these foods raw. Herbs and greens that contain good amounts of the B vitamins would include alfalfa, burdock, dandelion, fenugreek, parsley, sage, and watercress. Kelp is also high in B vitamins.

### Milk Replacements

Soy milk
Nut milks—seed milks
Wheat milk
Goat milk (bottled or canned evaporated)
Yogurt—thinned
Powdered whey (reconstituted)
Powdered milk
Buttermilk—powdered
Rice water—soaked, brought to boil, ground
   with liquid, and strained
Corn water—soaked, brought to boil, ground
   with liquid, and strained
Bean water—soaked, brought to boil, ground
   with liquid, and strained

Several recipes for milk replacements follow:

**Soy Milk**
Cornell Method—fortified

1 cup dry soybeans
6 cups boiling water plus 2 cups boil-
    ing water to heat blender
4 Tb. honey or 1 Tb. honey plus 3 Tb.
    barley malt extract
2 Tb. oil
1 Tb. calcium carbonate (1800 mg do-
    lomite)
1 tablet $B_{12}$ (25–50 mg)

Sort beans and soak from 2 to 16 hours in water to cover. The beans will double in bulk. Rinse and drain. Boil a large kettle of water.

Preheat blender with 2 cups boiling water. Empty blender and add 2 cups boiling water plus ⅓ of the beans. Grind thoroughly for 2 or 3 minutes. (Wrap a towel around the blender for insulation.)

Repeat until all beans have been ground.

Strain the beans and the water through a muslin or cheesecloth bag and squeeze to remove all the liquid. Measure the liquid.

Heat the soy milk in a saucepan placed over hot water for 30 minutes, uncovered. Stir occasionally to keep scum from forming on top. Add enough water to bring the amount of liquid back to the amount of liquid before heating.

Pour into bottles or jars after fortifying this way: For each batch of soy milk, add 25 to 50 micrograms of $B_{12}$, crushed. For each cup of soy milk add 1 tsp. safflower oil and ½ tsp. (300 milligrams) of calcium carbonate plus the sweetening agent of your choice to taste. Refrigerate.

Prep. time: 1 hour/soaking
time
1 cup dry beans makes 6–7 cups milk

Protein  ★ ★
Calcium  ★ ★

### No-Milk Beverages:

### Mandarin Shake

½ cup tofu,* drained well, crumbled,
   and chilled
¾ cup orange juice, chilled
2 ice cubes (optional)
Lemon juice to taste (optional)

* Tofu provides protein, iron, potassium.

Combine all ingredients in blender and blend until smooth. Serve immediately.

Prep. time: 10 minutes
Makes one regular or two tiny
servings.

Vitamin C   ★ ★
Protein   ★ ★ ★

### Sesame Milk

1 cup unhulled sesame seeds
4 cups water
1 Tb. honey

Toast seeds in 300° oven for 20 minutes. Combine half of the seeds with half of the water and honey in a blender and process for 2 minutes or until seeds are liquified. Strain through a large strainer, forcing as much water as possible from the mush. Discard mush and refrigerate milk. Use as a replacement for water or milk in cooked recipes, or combine with juices and fruits for delicious blender shakes.

Prep. time: 25 minutes
Yields 1 quart

Protein   ★ ★ ★
Calcium   ★ ★ ★ ★
Magnesium   ★ ★

### Easy Creamy Yogurt
(oven method)

>  6 cups powdered milk
>  1 10-oz. can evaporated skim milk
>  3 Tb. yogurt starter (or 3 Tb. plain
>     yogurt)
>  12 cups warm water

Mix all ingredients well and pour into clean jars. Set in a pot of very warm water. Cover the pot and place it in a prewarmed 200° oven. Turn off the oven and let it set 6 hours or overnight.

The advantage of this method is that no scalding is needed, and it can be made without special equipment. Keeps 5 days refrigerated.

Prep. time: 15 minutes      Protein   ★ ★ ★
Makes about 14 cups      Calcium   ★ ★ ★ ★

### No-Time-for-Breakfast Drink

>  2 cups skimmed or nondairy milk
>  1 Tb. safflower oil
>  2 Tb. barley malt extract
>  1 tsp. vanilla extract
>  1 heaping Tb. powdered brewer's
>     yeast
>  1 heaping Tb. granulated lecithin

Put all ingredients in blender and whip for 3 minutes. Refrigerate overnight. Shake well to mix in morning. Increase your use of the yeast and the lecithin gradually. Some use 4 Tb. of each!

Prep. time: 10 minutes      Protein   ★ ★ ★
Serves 2      Calcium   ★ ★ ★
                      B vitamins   ★ ★ ★ ★

### Samurai Special

½ cup tofu, well drained and crum-
    bled
½ cup unsweetened grape juice
1 Tb. lemon juice or to taste
½ banana, sliced
3–4 ice cubes

Combine all ingredients in blender and blend until
smooth, or until ice has dissolved. Serve immediately.

Prep. time: 10 minutes           **Protein**  ★ ★ ★
Makes one regular                **Vitamin C**  ★ ★
or two small serv-
ings.

### BREAKFAST

If you got up in time and thought ahead the day before, the
following breakfast ideas should stick to the ribs better:

### A-Little-Bit-of-Everything Cereal

3 cups cracked wheat
3 cups uncooked rolled oats
3 cups cornmeal
1½ cups brown rice
1½ cups bran
1 cup sesame seeds

Combine all ingredients and mix well. Store in airtight
canister and refrigerate. The night before, combine 1 cup
mix with 3 cups water. Soak overnight. Next morning, cook
in top of double boiler over simmering water for 10
minutes. Stir often. Serve in bowl with milk and honey, or
stir in applesauce to sweeten and cool it.

Prep. time: 5 minutes night      **Protein**  ★ ★
        before                   **Calcium**  ★ ★ ★ ★
        15 minutes in A.M.       **B vitamins**  ★ ★ ★ ★
Makes 4 servings                 **Magnesium**  ★ ★ ★ ★

### Super Sesame Oatmeal

1½ cups old-fashioned oats (not quick-
    cooking)
 3 cups water
 ½ tsp. salt
 1 Tb. butter
 ½ cup unhulled sesame seeds
 ½ cup plain yogurt
 ⅓ cup raisins

Bring oats and water to boil; cover and cook on low heat for
five minutes. Add other ingredients, stirring well.

| Prep. time: 10 minutes | Protein ★★★ | B vitamins ★★★ |
| Makes 4 generous | Calcium ★★★★ | Other: potassium |
| servings | Magnesium ★★★ | and iron |

### Granola

4 cups rolled oats
1 cup sesame seeds (unhulled)
1 cup sunflower seeds
1 cup chopped almonds
1 cup unsweetened coconut
1 cup wheat germ (or ½ cup wheat
  germ and ½ cup bran)
½ cup oil
1 cup raisins or dried fruit
½ cup honey
3 to 4 Tb. dolomite powder can be
  stirred into this, and no one will
  know the difference

Mix the first 6 ingredients with the oil in a large roasting
pan. Bake at 350° for about 30 minutes or until brown. Add
honey and raisins and toast a few minutes more. Cool and
store in tightly covered containers.

Prep. time: 45 minutes
Yields 10 to 12 cups

Protein   ★ ★ ★ ★
Calcium   ★ ★ ★ ★
Magnesium   ★ ★ ★ ★
B vitamins   ★ ★ ★ ★
Other:   iron and potassium

Coconut is a saturated fat, and since we are trying to cut down on honey, the following mixture might be preferred:

### Granola II

> 4 cups rolled oats
> 1 cup unsalted peanuts, chopped
> 1 cup sesame seeds (unhulled)
> 1 cup wheat germ
> 1 cup stone-ground whole wheat flour
> 1 cup nonfat milk powder
> ½ cup safflower oil
> 6 tsp. cinnamon
> 5 tsp. vanilla

Mix together all ingredients except the vanilla. Bake at 300° for 1 hour. Stir frequently. When done, sprinkle with vanilla. Mix. Cool. Serve in a bowl with unsweetened fruit juice poured over.

Prep. time: 1¼ hours
Makes 10 to 12 cups

Protein   ★ ★ ★ ★
Calcium   ★ ★ ★ ★
Magnesium   ★ ★ ★

B vitamins   ★ ★ ★ ★
Other:   iron and potassium

### River House Special Grits

> 1½ cups quick grits
> 6 cups water
> 1 lb. pasteurized cheese, cut into
>   small cubes
> ¾ cup butter or margarine
> 11 drops Tabasco sauce
> 3 eggs

Cook grits in water according to package directions. Remove from stove, add butter and cheese. Beat. Add Tabasco sauce. Beat in eggs. Bake in a large buttered casserole in preheated 375° oven for 1 hour.

Prep. time: 1½ hours        Protein  ★ ★ ★
Serves 12                Calcium  ★ ★ ★

If you really want to fill up your family for several hours, try the following variation on the basic pancake recipe. The dolomite powder contains calcium and magnesium; it should be helpful in calming the hyperactive child. The wheat germ and brewer's yeast are loaded with B vitamins, and the sausage and eggs, yogurt and wheat flour supply the protein to hold the blood sugar at an even level for three to five hours.

### Pancakes Plus

2 cups all-purpose dry ingredients
  mix (page 159)
¾ cup wheat germ
1 Tb. dolomite powder
2 cups plain yogurt
1 cup water
½ cup oil
3 eggs
1 lb. sausage
¼ cup brewer's yeast

Combine dry ingredients. Stir together yogurt, water, oil, and eggs and add to dry ingredients. Stir well. Set aside. Brown sausage. Drain off all fat but save 1 Tb. Stir in the 1 Tb. fat with ¼ cup brewer's yeast. Add to the mix and drop by ¼ cups onto lightly greased griddle. Turn when bubbles form and break on top; cook until brown. Careful what you put on top!

You can double the batch and freeze extras between

waxed paper layers. Toast the frozen ones in toaster for quick breakfasts.

| Prep. time: | Protein ★ ★ ★ ★ | B vitamins ★ ★ ★ ★ |
|---|---|---|
| 30 minutes | Calcium ★ ★ ★ ★ | Other: potassium, |
| Serves 6 to 8 | Magnesium ★ ★ ★ ★ | iron, and |
| | Vitamin A: fair | phosphorus |

### Yummy Baked Eggs

*For each serving:*

1 pat of butter
1 slice Swiss cheese (1 oz.)
1 egg
2 Tb. Parmesan cheese
Salt and pepper to taste

In an individual casserole dish place butter, Swiss cheese, broken egg, and Parmesan cheese in that order. Season lightly and bake covered for 10 to 12 minutes in preheated 350° oven.

Best served with some kind of fruit to balance the sodium of the cheese. Can be used at breakfast, lunch, or dinner.

| Prep. time: 12 minutes | Protein ★ ★ ★ ★ | Vitamin A ★ ★ ★ |
|---|---|---|
| Serves 1 | Calcium ★ ★ ★ ★ | B vitamins ★ ★ |
| | Magnesium ★ ★ ★ | |

Almost all the above baked goods can be enriched with dolomite powder, brewer's yeast, wheat germ, kelp powder, dessicated liver powder, and whatever else seems nourishing. The trick is to start slowly adding things to the mixtures so no one suspects. If your family finds out what you are doing, they may think you are playing tricks on them, and they will never trust you again.

### LUNCH OR SNACKS

Sandwiches are clever devices to carry good foods to the mouth and the stomach. If your family thinks that whole wheat breads are a poison, you may have to go slowly and sneak back the wheat germ the baker took out into the filling between the dull, white slices. Kids and adults love to build their own meal from time to time. A buffet gives them some options and makes them think they are in charge.

### High-Calcium Sandwich Fillings

1. To drained, skinned, and flaked salmon or mackerel, add mayonnaise and any of the following and mix well, then spread on slices of wholesome bread or stuff into pita bread:

| | |
|---|---|
| lemon juice | chopped onion |
| chopped egg | chopped pickle |
| chopped celery | chopped nuts |
| chopped parsley | |

Accompany with:

| | |
|---|---|
| cucumber rounds | alfalfa sprouts |
| lettuce | tomatoes |

2. To your favorite nut butter (peanut butter, almond butter, sesame butter, and the like), add any or all of the following and spread:

chopped dates
currants
raisins
chopped nuts—almonds, filberts, peanuts, Brazil nuts, and
   so on.
seeds—unhulled sesame seeds, sunflower seeds
apricot butter (see recipe)
bacon bits (if you can find bacon without sodium nitrite)
applesauce or crushed pineapple

3. With mashed leftover beans, put any of the following on sliced bread or stuff into pita bread:

chopped onion
sliced avocado
pepper rings
bacon bits (safe ones)
chopped nuts
chili powder

sliced tomato
lettuce leaves
cucumber slices
chopped parsley
sliced radishes

4. To a chopped, mashed hard-cooked egg add mayonnaise and any of the following and spread on bread:

chopped onion
chopped parsley
chopped green pepper
chopped celery

chopped pickle
chopped nuts
garlic powder
paprika (pinch)

5. Spread a slice of bread with mayonnaise. Add a slice of sweet and tangy meat loaf and accompany with any of the following, and top with a second slice of bread.

tomato slices
pickles
lettuce

avocado slices
onion slices
green pepper rings

6. Use falafel or fish patties (see recipes) between buns, slices of bread, or stuffed into pita bread along with:

mayonnaise

hummus (pureed chick
  peas and garlic)
avocado slices
tabooli (see p. 232)
tomato slices

lemony beans
  (see recipe)
chopped parsley
shredded lettuce
onion rings
hot sauce

7. Use herbs and seeds for extra calcium:

poppy seed—41 mg/Tb.
celery seed—35 mg/Tb.
dill—32 mg/Tb.

cinnamon—28 mg/Tb.
thyme—26 mg/Tb.
fennel—24 mg/Tb.

**7.** Use herbs and seeds for extra calcium: (*cont'd.*)

savory—30 mg/Tb.
basil—30 mg/Tb.

oregano—24 mg/Tb.
terragano—18 mg/Tb.

Every little bit adds up.

### Peanut Butter Spread

1 cup peanut butter, natural style
¼ cup toasted sunflower seeds,
    shelled, or unhulled sesame seeds
½ cup chopped dried fruit
2 Tb. applesauce, unsweetened
1 Tb. brewer's yeast
1 Tb. dolomite, bone meal, or cal-
    cium lactate powder
1 tsp. orange juice

Mix all ingredients in blender until desired consistency is reached and refrigerate.

Prep. time: 10 minutes
Yield: 2 cups

Protein ★★★★    B vitamins ★★★
Calcium ★★★    Other: potassium

### Sesame Butter

1½ cups unhulled sesame seeds
¼ cup sesame, safflower, or vegeta-
    ble oil
1 Tb. honey (optional)

Place sesame seeds in a shallow pan and roast at 300° for 20 minutes. Cool, then pour into blender jar. Blend, covered, on medium speed until seeds are ground into meal. Add the oil slowly, blending and stirring until creamy. Blend in honey if desired.

Prep. time: 30 minutes
Yield: 1½ cups

Protein ★★★★    B vitamins ★★★
Calcium ★★★★    Magnesium ★★★

### High-Protein Cheese Spread

1 lb. Colby cheese, grated
8 oz. muenster cheese, grated
8 oz. medium or sharp cheddar
   cheese, grated
1 cup plain yogurt
1 cup toasted or raw wheat germ
1 Tb. onion juice
½ tsp. salt
⅛ tsp. red pepper
1 cup sunflower seeds, shelled

Place cheeses in mixer or food processor. Mix or blend until cheese starts to hold together. Add yogurt and mix well. Stir in remaining ingredients except sunflower seeds, mixing to blend. Stir in sunflower seeds by hand. Chill. Serve as a sandwich filling with lots of alfalfa sprouts, or stuff into celery. Keeps well in refrigerator for 2 to 3 weeks. Recipe may be halved.

| Prep. time: | Protein ★ ★ ★ ★ | B vitamins ★ ★ ★ ★ |
|---|---|---|
| 20 minutes | Calcium ★ ★ ★ ★ | Other: potassium, |
| Yield: 5½ cups | Magnesium ★ ★ ★ | phosphorus, and iron |

### Curried Snack Mix

1 8-oz. package natural-style corn
   chips
1 cup whole or broken walnuts
1 cup whole or broken pecans
2 qts. freshly popped corn
¼ lb. butter or margarine
1½ tsp. garlic salt
1 tsp. curry powder
½ tsp. salt
2 dashes Tabasco sauce

Mix first 4 ingredients in a large bowl. Melt the butter or margarine in a small saucepan and add the remaining ingredients. Drizzle the butter mixture onto the popcorn and nuts. Stir until the seasonings are mixed well. Bake in preheated 300° oven for 30 minutes, stirring every 10 minutes. Cool and store in tightly covered containers.

Prep. time:     Protein  ★ ★ ★          B vitamins  ★ ★ ★
40 minutes      Magnesium  ★ ★ ★ ★      Other:  phosphorus
Yield: 5 quarts Vitamin A  ★ ★ ★

### Zorba's Delight

20 almonds raw, finely chopped or
   grated
½ cup orange or apple juice
3 large dried figs, stemmed and
   chopped
2-inch slice of banana (optional)
3 or 4 ice cubes

Chop or grate almonds in blender. With spatula, push fragments off sides and back into bottom of blender. Add remaining ingredients and blend until ice dissolves. Drink while cool.

Prep. time:     Protein  ★ ★ ★         Other:  potassium
10 minutes      Calcium  ★ ★ ★                 and
Serves 2        Magnesium  ★ ★ ★ ★             phosphorus
                B vitamins  ★ ★ ★

### Tortilla Chips

6 corn tortillas
Salt (sea salt, if possible)

Preheat oven to 400°. Cut each tortilla into 6 pie-shaped pieces. Spread on cookie sheet and salt lightly. Bake for 10 minutes. Remove from oven and turn each one over; return to oven for 3 minutes more. Cool.

Prep. time: 15 minutes
Yield: 2 cups

Use the recipe above to get the following dip to the mouth.

### Guacamole

4 medium-size avocados, pitted and
  peeled
2 Tb. sour cream
1 tsp. garlic salt or minced garlic
Dash salt and pepper
Juice of 1 lemon
½ tomato, chopped

Mash avocados, blend in sour cream; add garlic salt and salt
and pepper. Add lemon juice. Stir in tomato and serve with
tortilla chips.

Prep. time: 10 minutes         **Magnesium** ★ ★ ★
Serves 8                       **Other:** potassium


### Nachos

Tortilla chips
½ lb. cheddar cheese, grated
½ lb. (Monterey) jack cheese, grated
1 tomato, cut up
4 green onions, chopped
1 3½-oz. can jalapeño peppers (optional)

Spread tortilla chips on cookie sheet. Top with both
cheeses and sprinkle the tomatoes and onions on top. Dot
with peppers if used. Bake in preheated 350° oven until
cheese is melted. Serve hot.

Prep. time: ½ hour            **Protein** ★ ★ ★
Serves 4                      **Calcium** ★ ★ ★ ★


### MAIN DISHES

Use this as a basis of soup stock or as added water in
any vegetable or meat casserole. Freeze in ice trays; use
cubes when steaming vegetables.

### Soup Stock

2-3 lbs. of bones, preferably cracked
1 to 2 quarts water, to cover
2 Tb. vinegar per quart of water
1 onion, quartered
Celery tops

Boil bones gently in water until meat falls off. Remove bones and scrape marrow out. Add marrow to stock; stir well. Strain.

Prep. time: 2 hours
Yield: 1 to 2 quarts stock

Protein ★★
Calcium ★★★★
Magnesium ★★

Beans are full of protein and B vitamins, and they can taste good. Try to get the family used to legumes as a source of protein. They are good in amino-acid quality, have no fat, and are cheaper than meat.

### Tangy Lima Beans

1 large onion, chopped
1 clove garlic, chopped fine
2 Tb. oil
Salt and pepper
2 cups lima beans (1 16-oz. can)
1 (heaping) Tb. whole wheat flour
2 Tb. wine vinegar

In a large skillet sauté onion and garlic until soft and yellow. Add drained lima beans and vinegar. Save that liquid from the beans! Mix. Sprinkle on the flour while stirring to make a sauce. Add some of the liquid from the bean can if the mixture looks too dry. Mix well. Season, mix again, and serve. Use as a side dish; double the recipe if a main dish.

Prep. time: 30 minutes
Serves 3 or 4 as a side dish

Protein ★★★
B vitamins ★★★

### Spaghetti

1½ lb. ground beef
1 onion, diced
¼ tsp. garlic powder
¼ cup brewer's yeast
2 15-oz. cans tomato sauce
2 Tb. Italian seasoning
1 tsp. salt
½ tsp. pepper
2 Tb. honey
8-oz. package whole wheat spaghetti
1 cup grated Parmesan cheese
1 cup grated Swiss cheese

Brown beef with onion and garlic powder; do not drain. Stir in yeast and tomato sauce; bring to boil over medium-high heat. Add seasonings and honey. Cover and reduce heat; simmer 30 minutes. Uncover and simmer 20 more minutes. Meanwhile prepare spaghetti according to package directions. Drain well and place in a large ovenproof dish. Top with sauce, then add cheeses. Place under broiler for 2 minutes, until cheese melts.

Prep. time: 1½ hours  **Protein**  ★ ★ ★ ★   **B vitamins**  ★ ★ ★ ★
Serves 8  **Calcium**  ★ ★ ★ ★   **Other:  phosphorus**
  **Magnesium**  ★ ★ ★

 

There is some potassium in the eggplant, but this should be eaten with other food high in potassium to help balance the sodium in the cheeses. For example, serve with dried fruits or nuts or maybe a bran muffin. One to 2 Tb. of brewer's yeast could be added to the cooked dish, and that would neutralize the sodium.

Eggplant has lots of fiber. Its versatility makes it an attractive ingredient in a variety of dishes.

### Eggplant-Rice Combo

    1 cup brown rice
    2½ cups water
    2 Tb. butter
    ½ tsp. salt
    1 eggplant, pared
    ½ cup chopped onion
    1 cup grated Swiss cheese
    1 cup Parmesan cheese
Seasoning (such as fine herbs)

Cook rice in water with butter and salt for 45 to 50 minutes until done. Cook eggplant, covered, until tender; drain well and add onion. Preheat oven to 400°. Place eggplant mixture in blender; blend until smooth. Add this to cooked rice. Next add the cheese and seasonings. Stir well; cover for a few minutes, until the cheese has melted. Transfer to a casserole, cover, and heat in oven for 10 minutes. Serve hot.

Prep. time: 1 hour      Protein  ★ ★ ★ ★      Vitamin A  ★ ★
Yield: 6 servings        Calcium  ★ ★ ★ ★      B vitamins  ★ ★ ★ ★
                         Magnesium  ★ ★        Other: phosphorus


### Easy Quiche

    4 eggs
    1½ cups plain yogurt
    1 Tb. soy flour
    ½ tsp. salt
    ¼ tsp. pepper
    ¼ tsp. onion salt
    1 medium onion, cut in chunks
    1½ cups Swiss cheese, cut in
        chunks
    1 lb. sausage, browned until done
    1 9-inch unbaked whole-grain pie
        shell

Place first 6 ingredients in blender and process on low speed until blended thoroughly. Stop blender and add onions and cheese. Process on high speed long enough to chop and distribute ingredients evenly. Place sausage on the bottom of the pie crust and pour blended mixture over it. Bake in preheated 375° oven for 35 to 45 minutes, until a knife inserted in the center comes out clean.

Prep. time: 1 hour    **Protein** ★★★★    **B vitamins** ★★★
Serves 4 to 6    **Calcium** ★★★★    **Other:** phosphorus
   **Magnesium** ★★

### Zucchini Casserole

    1 cup brown rice
    2 medium onions, diced
    1 medium green pepper, diced
    3 medium zucchini, sliced thin
    2 Tb. safflower oil
    3 tomatoes, chopped
    2 Tb. vinegar
    ½ cup salt-free tomato or V-8 juice
    ½ tsp. black pepper
     2 tsp. onion powder or minced fresh
    ⅛ tsp. garlic powder or minced fresh
    ½ tsp. ground horseradish
    2–3 Tb. brewer's yeast

Sauté onion, green pepper, and rice in oil until rice is dark brown. Add all the other ingredients. Simmer 5 minutes. Put in casserole. Bake at 350° for 30 minutes.

Prep. time: 50 minutes    **Vitamin A** ★★
Serves 6    **B vitamins** ★★★★
   **Vitamin C** ★★

### Squash au Gratin

1 lb. summer squash
¼ cup milk
1 cup grated cheddar cheese
Salt and pepper to taste

Wash and remove the stems of the squash. Cut into quarters. Cook in saucepan with water until soft. Drain. Mash. Add milk and seasoning. Put into casserole. Mix 3 Tb. of cheese into squash. Sprinkle the rest on the top. Bake until cheese melts. This is a good way to use up squash or zucchini. Most everything is good with cheese.

Prep. time: 45 minutes
Serves 6

Protein  ★★
Calcium  ★★★★
Vitamin A  ★★

### BREADS

Use in your favorite quick-mix recipes for muffins, pancakes, waffles, quick breads, biscuits, etc. No preservatives and, pro-rated, little sugar.

### Quick-Mix All-Purpose Wheat Mix (see also p. 159)

6 cups whole wheat
3 cups all-purpose unbleached flour
1½ cups instant nonfat dry milk
1 Tb. salt (sea salt preferred)
1 cup sugar—use less as time goes
  by
½ cup wheat germ
¼ cup baking powder
2 cups vegetable shortening

Thoroughly mix all dry ingredients in a large bowl. Cut in shortening with a pastry blender until there are no lumps. Put in a large airtight container and store in a cool, dry place.

Prep. time: 30 minutes
13 cups

Calcium  ★★
B vitamins  ★★

### Refrigerator Bran Rolls

1 cup boiling water
1 cup unprocessed bran
¾ cup butter or margarine
2 beaten eggs, at room temperature
1 pkg. yeast
¼ tsp. salt
1 cup warm water
1 cup whole wheat flour
4 cups unbleached flour

Combine boiling water, bran, butter or margarine, and honey. Stir, remove from heat, and cool for a few minutes until lukewarm; add beaten eggs. Stir together yeast, salt, and whole wheat flour. Add warm water and mix on low speed for 1 minute. Add bran mixture and 2 cups unbleached flour. Place in mixer and blend on low speed, then on medium speed for 2 minutes. Stir in remaining flour; mix well. Cover and refrigerate overnight or for up to 5 days.

To form rolls, punch dough down and form in a well-greased pan. Allow to rise covered for 2 hours. Bake in preheated 350° oven for 20 to 25 minutes.

Prep. time: 30 minutes/over-
　　　　　night
Yield:　2 9-inch pans of rolls,
　　　　13–16 rolls each pan

Protein  ★ ★ ★
Calcium  ★ ★
Magnesium  ★ ★ ★ ★
Vitamin A  ★ ★
B vitamins  ★ ★ ★ ★
Other:  phosphorus, iron,
　　　　and potassium

### Animal Crackers

1 cup sunflower seeds, shelled
½ cup wheat germ, unsweetened co-
    conut, or cornmeal
1 Tb. honey
Dash salt
¼ cup cold water

Grind sunflower seeds to a coarse meal texture in blender.
Remove to a mixing bowl; add wheat germ, honey, and salt
and water. Stir with a fork until blended, then place on a
lightly greased cookie sheet. Cover with waxed paper and
roll to ⅛- to ¼-inch thickness. Remove paper and cut with
animal-shaped cookie cutter or into other desired shapes
(or score into squares) and bake in preheated 300° oven for
15 to 20 minutes, until lightly browned. Cool for 5 minutes,
then remove to wire racks to finish drying. Use as snacks or
as meal accompaniments. *Tip:* Bake dough scraps with
crackers; use as casserole toppings, fillings, or breading.

Prep. time: 30 minutes
Yield: 2 to 4 dozen crackers

Protein ★ ★ ★
Calcium ★ ★ ★ ★
Magnesium ★ ★ ★
B vitamins ★ ★ ★
Other:  phosphorus, iron,
        and potassium

### Wheat-Germ Bread

5½ to 6½ cups unsifted stone-ground
    whole wheat flour, divided
2 pkg. dry yeast
1½ cups nonfat milk
½ cup water
½ cup salt-free butter or safflower oil
1 egg yolk
1 whole egg
1½ cups wheat germ
1 Tb. wheat germ
1 egg white, beaten

In large mixing bowl mix together 3 cups flour and the yeast. In saucepan heat milk, water, and butter or oil until warm. Add to flour mixture. Add egg and yolk. Mix at low speed until moistened. Beat 3 minutes at medium speed. By hand, gradually stir in wheat germ and enough remaining flour to make a soft dough.

Knead on floured surface until smooth and elastic (about 20 minutes). Place in bowl rubbed with safflower oil, turning dough to oil top. Cover. Let rise in warm place until light and doubled (about 1 hour). Punch down dough.

Divide into 2 parts. Roll or pat each portion on lightly floured surface into a 12 by 8-inch rectangle. Cut each rectangle into 2 equal 4 by 12-inch strips. Pinch edges of each strip together to make a rope. Twist 2 ropes around each other. Seal ends and tuck under loaf.

Place in well-oiled loaf pan. Cover, let rise 30 to 40 minutes. Lightly brush with beaten egg white. Sprinkle with additional wheat germ. Bake at 350° for 35 to 45 minutes. Cover with foil last 5 to 10 minutes of baking.

This is a heavy, thick, delicious bread. For a lighter bread use only ¾ cup wheat germ.

Prep. time: 1½ hours plus          **Protein**   ★ ★
              45 minutes baking time   **B vitamins**   ★ ★ ★ ★
Yield: 2 loaves

### Whole-Grain Pocket Bread

4¾ cups whole wheat or unbleached
   flour
 1 pkg. yeast
1½ tsp. salt
1¾ cups sesame milk
 2 Tb. oil
 1 Tb. honey

Combine 2 cups flour, yeast, and salt. Heat sesame milk, oil, and honey together until liquids are very warm but not boiling. Cool slightly and add to yeast mixture. Blend, then beat on medium speed for 2 minutes. Add remaining flour and mix well, then beat on high speed 2 to 3 minutes. Let dough rest, covered, for 20 minutes.

Divide dough into 18 parts, shaping each part into a smooth ball. Cover and let rise 30 minutes. Roll each ball into a 4- to 5-inch-wide circle. Place on wire racks and bake 4 to 6 at a time (depending on size of racks) in preheated 500° oven for about 4 minutes, until puffy and toasted on top. Remove immediately and cool for 1 minute on wire rack; then cut into halves with sharp serrated knife, separating top from bottom. When cool, stuff with sandwich filling as desired. Sausage and egg stuffing makes a quick nutritious breakfast.

Prep. time: 1½ hours   **Protein**  ★ ★ ★       **B vitamins**  ★ ★ ★
Yield: 36                    **Calcium**  ★ ★ ★ ★   **Other:**  **Iron and**
                             **Magnesium**  ★ ★ ★              **phosphorus**

# Sugar Cravings, 10 Foods, and Moods

Some crave carbohydrates, and the sweeter the better. Most of us like or even love sweets, but certain children crave sugar. They have to have sugar on their pre-sweetened cereal. They have to have ice cream (20 percent sugar) daily; some can eat quarts or a gallon a day—and stay thin.

Their desire for sweet, soft foods seems to be so strong that a salad or a vegetable is considered poison. Many of them have a nose full of phlegm and so are unable to chew for more than a few seconds. Chewing finely ground hamburger is about all they can tolerate. Pies, cakes, chocolates, jam, sweet rolls, marshmallows, jelly beans, pop, and cola drinks are daily favorites. They will steal money to get a sweet fix. They can sometimes be caught in the middle of the night eating a whole box of brown sugar. They always put too much syrup on their pancakes.

Glucose-tolerance tests show that most of these

141

sugar-cravers have abnormal responses to sugar ingestion. Their blood sugars would rise very high and then drop off to very low levels. Some sugar levels would drop right off without the early rise. But some had normal rises and falls, so the blood test was not a specific for all sugar-cravers.

The amount of food these children scarf down would make most people gain a pound an hour. The love of sweet, rich food suggests low or falling blood sugar, and the lack of gain has to mean some problem with absorption once the food arrives in the intestinal tract. Indeed, many therapists use pancreatic enzymes with meals to help food digestion and absorption.

The overconsumption of naked carbohydrates tells us that these children are below normal in their consumption of B vitamins. B vitamins are essential for the metabolism of all foods. Once the body gets behind in the supply of B vitamins, the intestinal enzymes cannot function optimally. Poor absorption and the feeling of hunger are indicators that the body needs B vitamins.

Foods rich in all the Bs, especially $B_3$, would be important, but vitamin B complex in concentrated form (capsules or injections) may be necessary before foods themselves could be wholly relied on.

Complex carbohydrates (nuts, seeds, vegetables, and some fruits) are best, since they keep the blood sugar more even and contain B complex vitamins. In three weeks many parents say "He's eating half as much food and gaining weight"—which must mean an absorption problem was part of the craving problem.

Almost all such children become restless, irritable, surly or frankly hyperactive within half an hour to two hours after the sugar ingestion. But not all. So sugar ingestion was not the universal answer.

Not all ticklish children are hyperactive, and not all children who crave sugar become hyperactive. There is a good chance, however, that a child who is sensitive and craves and eats sugar will be likely to be a school problem.

To avoid the trauma of blood tests, I needed to find some observable behavior or physical sign that was palpable enough for parent, teacher, or neighbor to note easily. (The supermarket clerk can spot these children because they cannot leave the displays alone.)

Going down a list of questions asked of parents of children with school-related problems, there were three or four related questions that all seemed to answer affirmatively:

> Is he a Jekyll-and-Hyde type of person?
> Does he have mood swings?
> Is he terrible-tempered Mr. Bang?
> Is he emotionally unstable?
> Does he fly into rages for no good reason?
> Does the teacher report good and bad days?

We all have mood swings, but these children *really* have mood swings and from the slightest provocation. You say "Good morning, Charlie," and Charlie pulls a knife. One day Eddie can read from the book, and the very next day nothing comes out of his mouth. You know he can do it as he did it just twenty-four hours before. Is he sick, stubborn, having an attack? "Inconsistent work" is what the teacher would put on the report card. "He cannot work up to his ability." "Unable to finish what he starts." "Goof-off" is what she would like to say about Eddie, but that's pejorative.

I knew about these wild, impulsive, mean, uncontrollable children who grew up to become mean, wild, antisocial adults. These are the children (and adults) who can be sweet, pleasant, compliant, thoughtful, caring, loving, following the ten commandments one minute, hour, or day, and then for no obvious or valid reason become depressed, moody, mean, crabby, bitter, surly, aggressive, crude the next. Some therapists figured they were the product of inconsistent discipline, but since the advent of psychosurgery it was felt that a neurological reverberative circuit near the mean (limbic) part of the animal brain sent out electrical impulses occasionally and the animal brain took over—like a seizure. I used to have electroencephalograms done on these patients, and the neurologist usually was able to find some little extra brainwave that suggested an abnormal discharge from the lower brain. All very mysterious, but at least we had something to point to. And there were medicines that were almost specific for the problem. Phenobarbital usually stimulated them. Dilantin (R) (phenytoin) seemed to have a modifying effect on these children's highs and lows; they still had them, but the intensity was not so great. After a few months, most of the children could be taken off the medicine and the benefits would continue.

I now feel certain that I was treating a symptom, but I was not discovering the cause of the outbursts. If someone has seizures or epilepsy, he should be having fits all the time. There has to be a reason why he is "good" for hours or weeks and then "bad" for seconds or minutes. Some neurobiochemical phenomenon allowed some irritable focus to spread to another area of the brain, and then that part of the brain responsible for the antisocial act (e.g., kicking a foot through the wall) would take over. One had to assume that a behavior was built in but dormant in the lower animal center, the limbic system. When social control (in the neocortex, the higher human area of the brain) is lost or ineffective, for a variety of reasons, the lower, savage, antisocial behavior surfaces.

Enough research has been done on the nervous system to provide a working hypothesis to explain these fluctuations in mood and thought. Even a superficial understanding of the metabolism of the brain makes changes in mood and behavior readily understandable. The brain is a very busy organ; it is the busiest organ we have. (The liver and kidneys vie for second place.) A fourth of the blood volume ejected from the heart at every beat goes to the brain. The brain has no storage for energy. The muscles have stored glycogen, but it is only available for the muscles. The liver has enough glycogen stored for about an ordinary day's needs. The child's brain has about two to three times the energy needs of the adult brain.

If, then, the supply of oxygen, glucose, water, vitamins, minerals, and amino acids is inadequate for even a short period of time, important social, cognitive, and perceptive areas of the brain will not function optimally and the lower centers will take over. These lower centers have only phylogenetically built-in responses such as rage, depression, excessive activity (or hypoactivity), hunger, sex, somnolence, or other variables of the flight-or-fight response. There is nothing psychological or learned in these animal responses; these areas that "turn on" in the limbic system are organized emotional nerve centers that we social animals need at appropriate times. It is the inappropriateness of the responses, the utter lack of control that is the key. (Your six-year-old does not like oatmeal, so he dumps it on the floor. That is inappropriate in my house.)

Therefore, we cannot let the blood sugar (or oxygen, or water) slip down too low or too rapidly, for cortical functions will be compromised; the little lights will go out, and the devil in all of us takes over. (A wife does not recognize her husband at breakfast time because her blood sugar is too low. She *has* to have a bowl of ice cream while watching the 11 P.M. news. She makes too much insulin in response to the rapid rise of glucose in her bloodstream from the ice cream, and by morning the part of the cortex of the brain that has the "recognition of spouse" area is not energized sufficiently to give the rest of her brain any clue as to the identity of this man sitting across the table. "Who is this guy?" she mutters half-aloud. Once given insight, the husband that night knocks the sugary mess out of her hands and forces twenty almonds down her throat. The next morning she awakens and immediately identifies her next of kin. "John! It's nice to know the guy you married is the guy you're sleeping with.")

Mothers report their children are more compliant after meals than on an empty stomach. Children will not poison themselves with drugs at 4:30 P.M. if they have a protein snack at 3:00 P.M. Notice how crazy your children are if you make them wait for Thanksgiving dinner from breakfast time; "save your appetite" is the best way to lose your sanity. The child who is rewarded with a sweet snack if he will just "go to bed" is usually the one who takes an hour to dress in the morning. He sits naked on the floor staring at his sock, wondering what to do with it. "Yeah, I'm almost dressed" is his response when told to hurry or he will be late. He is functioning on about one-third of his usual brain circuits.

One can see how blood sugar fluctuations can trigger some seizures. The wild rage attacks that I thought were all due to abnormal brain waves years ago may really have blood-sugar fluctuations as the basis. The odd brainwave may be a reality, but it is now known that a significant number of EEGs are different when taken on a full or empty stomach. Dr. William Philpott of Oklahoma City feels that a large number of people with epilepsy do not have true epilepsy but a carbohydrate dysfunction that allows brainwaves to change (or there is a change in acid-base balance) which in susceptible people allows them to have seizures. The drugs used raise the threshold for nerve-cell discharge, so they are helpful, but would it not be more scientific to improve the basic biochemistry of the whole body?

Work with prisoners and juvenile delinquents indicates that a fair share of crime has a biochemical more than a sociological or psychological basis. Over 60 percent of prisoners have abnormal glucose-tolerance test results. Seventy-five percent of prisoners were hyperactive children. If juvenile offenders are put on probation, many do not return to crime. If they are also taken off pop and sweets, twice as many do not get into trouble again, reports Barbara Reed, a probation officer in Cuyahoga Falls, Ohio. Alexander Schauss has verified the nutrition connection with crime (see his book, *Diet, Crime, and Deliquency*).

But lots of people who eat improperly never get into trouble or get sick, and lots of people who eat all the proper foods are in trouble all the time, either with the police or with bacteria. Of course, that is the delight but also the frustration of dealing with humans. No one rule fits all people. The causes of sickness and sociopathy are multifactoral. Just when we think we have a fact nailed down, forever a truism, some new research comes along to discredit it.

The two factors I notice in almost every case of maladaption in home, school, and peer relations are exquisite sensitivity to everything in the environment and the Jekyll-and-Hyde response to inappropriate foods. Maybe if the ticklish ones were fed properly, their brains could process all the incoming stimuli without noticing the overload. Maybe if we could educate the Jekyll-and-Hyde types never to eat sugar and to nibble on some good food every two to three hours, their bodies would not overproduce the insulin. It would be a start.

Young students will often believe their teachers more readily than they do their parents. Teachers, aware of this power, must use it to indoctrinate children with the concept that *no child who did not bring his or her brain to school can learn anything.* Until they get locked into the idea, the teacher must ask each pupil daily "What did you eat for breakfast?" If the answer is "boxed cereal and pop," he is sent home for a proper meal. If he doesn't remember, his brain is already gone for that day, and if he is sent home, he may not find it.

The important diet change to control the Jekyll-and-Hyde symptoms would be to allow no quick sugars (white or brown sugar, corn syrup, maple syrup, molasses or honey) in the house, although many carbo addicts will have to have decreasing amounts of honey or fructose for three months.

If the personality alters and sugar has not been consumed, a record of all foods ingested in the previous two to twelve hours must be made. As time passes it will become obvious what food is the culprit. A partial fast may help. Testing the saliva pH may be revealing. (For a more detailed explanation of the saliva test, see pages 212–213.)

### Questions and Answers

**Q. I really have a crabby, disagreeable child. He is now two years old and is never satisfied. Everything must go his way. He needs to win. It's "mine, mine" or "gimme, gimme." I wanted and loved him and nursed him. He won't eat what's on his plate. He craves sweets. He says "yuk" when he sees a vegetable. I'm getting to dislike him although I love him.**

**A.** The two-year-old is supposed to be noncompliant, as if practicing for adolescence, but he is cheerful about it more often than he is glum. If a baby (person) laughs and smiles more than he cries and frowns, it suggests he is doing OK. If he seems unhappy most of the time, he may not be feeling well. There may be some attention-getting reward system operating that reinforces this unacceptable performance. You are supposed to turn your back on it. I assume he has had a checkup to rule out infections, anemia, or allergies and that you have treated for worms.

If, however, he has peaks of acceptable, loving behavior and then plunges into the valley of surliness, quickly write down what he ate—or didn't—for the two to twelve hours prior to the glumpy time. After a few of these you will be able to see a pattern. I can become miserable with a headache and poutiness if I am out in the sun and eat a red hot dog, a serving of potato salad, and one ear of corn and have half a can of beer. It usually takes all five of these poisons working in concert to put me down.

It doesn't have to be sugar. It could be the onset of an infection, premenstrual tension, coloring in vitamins, the odor of mint blowing from a nearby field. If it is a food, it is usually the child's favorite. If he loves toast, you can bet he is allergic and addicted to wheat.

**Q. My three-year-old is a little hyper and gets really wild when he eats sugar but, in general, does OK. His nursery-school teacher says he is doing well, has friends, and an even personality. But when I get him he is wild-eyed, demanding, restless, wound up. Is he responding to me?**

A. He might be. Try to turn your back on these antics, which helps defuse them. It may be the normal explosion of pent-up energies and frustrations built up by the social pressures of school to conform. They need a period after school to rant and rave. Use the Haim Ginott technique: "Say, you're really burned." Or "Wow, you seem upset today." Hyper kids are more extreme, and a poor diet makes it worse. But we all need some outlet and a sympathetic ear.

But just in case, find out what the snacks are just before you pick him up. Some protein and calcium about a half hour before your arrival (for both of you) might just make your relationship calmer and more rewarding.

**Q. My five-year-old is loud, irritating, and thoughtless after sugar, food color, dairy products—all the things served at parties. He is getting fewer invitations to parties**

because he is a less-than-satisfactory guest. How do I help
his social life?

A. You can call ahead in the hope that the hostess
will provide safe snacks, or you may bring along your own
safe cake and explain why. But children do not like to
appear different from their peer group. An allergic reaction
can be assuaged with the preventative ingestion of vitamin
C (500 to 2000 mg), calcium (500 to 1000 mg), and $B_6$ (100
mg). If you could get these and a protein snack down him
about thirty to sixty minutes before the party, he should be
calmer, and if he *does* eat an allergen or some naked
carbohydrate, it would not be enough to cause symptoms.
Developing social skills is as important as learning good
eating habits.

Q. Our fourteen-year-old daughter can be sweet,
bright, thoughtful, and a real joy when she wants to, but in
this last year she has been having some mood swings that
make me wonder what sort of a witch I have reared. Do all
adolescents have to act so awful?

A. Teenagers use their parents to test life styles.
They are struggling with their own feelings of independ-
ence-dependence. They grow fast and are usually raven-
ously hungry all the time. What they eat can have a
palpable effect on their behavior. Everything that goes in
should be as nourishing as possible. Because you cannot
monitor every morsel, it would be smart to provide extra
calcium as well as B, C, D, and A vitamins in the food plus
an all-purpose vitamin and mineral capsule containing the
daily recommended doses of each. Ask your doctor.

We are all different, and since adolescence is such a
strain, try to read her body for clues that would indicate
what system is most vulnerable.

If she has insomnia or muscle and menstrual cramps,
push the calcium, magnesium, and vitamin D. If her low
point is related to her periods, use extra B vitamins,
especially vitamin $B_6$.

If her skin is pimply, consider zinc foods, but if her flow is heavy and her upper arms and thighs feel rough, maybe vitamin A and foods containing it would help.

If she is allergic and frequently ill, a bigger dose of vitamin C and C-bearing foods should help.

If she is gaining weight and has stopped growing, check her eating habits. Nibbling good food six times a day is the best way to maintain weight as well as lose it if necessary.

Once the nutrition is as optimal as possible, try to do some domestic psychology. If she has friends, laughs more than cries, and is working at her appropriate grade level, she is doing OK.

If she gets mononucleosis, something went wrong.

**Q. I'm afraid to say no to my fifteen-month-old. Three months ago he had febrile convulsions associated with roseola. Now when he is crossed and has a temper tantrum, he holds his breath, turns blue, his eyes roll up, and he passes out. I'm really scared of these, but I don't want him to get spoiled.**

**A.** If you can believe me, these spells do not hurt him unless he falls on something. They are not a form of epilepsy. The tantrums are a normal communication response for this age, but the progression on to the spell suggests low blood sugar, a calcium deficiency, or a need for $B_6$. See if there is a correlation between them and his feeling punk because of something he ate one to six hours previously.

By the time you figure out what it is due to and what extra nutrients he needs, he will have outgrown them.

**Q. I know I am a crabby bitch for the few days before my period, but my husband is a jerk then also. My son, age six years, is nice most of the time but seems to know my bad days because then he talks louder and slams doors and is surly. If they were better, I would be OK.**

**A.** Menstruation is a stress, and stress makes the

blood sugar drop. Allergies surface, fluids accumulate, headaches appear. You are unable to keep the world at a comfortable distance. Your enzymes are not getting enough B complex vitamins. Your pleasant, social brain is bombarded with too many unignorable stimuli at the very time it is least able to handle them because of the low blood sugar and swollen tissue. Self-control is shot. Many women resort to binging on chocolate and other sweets.

Once your social brain is on tilt, you have no insight to take remedial action. You should be on the nibbling diet all the time as a preventative (no quick carbohydrates), and be consuming extra B complex all the time and extra $B_6$ at the critical times (i.e., just before and during your period).

**Q. My son does well in school except for math and social studies. The teacher says she knows he can do it, but it never gets down on paper so she can grade him. He starts out fine in the morning for history, English, and gym, but math and social studies are in the afternoon, and he can't hack them.**

**A.** That off-and-on, up-and-down, inconsistent performance is the giveaway that his diet is responsible. Maybe exercise burns up so many calories that his blood sugar is so low he has to eat some quick carbohydrate. Then he overproduces insulin, his blood sugar falls rapidly, and the math and social studies departments of his brain become nonoperative.

You have to make sure he is off the sugar and junk (white flour and quick carbohydrates) and get him to eat a lunch that will sustain him longer. Or send a note so he can eat nuts and cheese in the class. (For the teacher to allow that, you may have to furnish snacks for the whole class! In some parts of the country, this can be tax deductible.)

However, it can be something to which he is allergic, usually a favorite food. Wheat as in sandwiches, corn, beef, milk, potatoes. Anything can do anything. The chemicals in the drinking water can upset some. Get him to experiment to see if he can read his own body and tell *you*. Get him to test his own salivary acidity with pH paper. See if he can correlate the way he feels with the acidity or alkalinity of the saliva.

### High-Protein Recipes

The most commonly accepted superior source of complete protein is meat, including poultry. However, soy grits contain the highest concentration of protein, per weight, of any food. However, soy is not a complete protein and must be combined with other sources. Grits can be added to breads, made into pilafs or puddings, and used in any number of creative ways—and they are a more economical buy than meat.

Other foods high in protein include cheeses, wheat germ, and nut butters. Nuts and seeds, fish, eggs, grains and legumes, soy flour and sprouts are also excellent sources of protein.

Most children in our country are not protein-deficient. If there is a fault, it is in the timing. It seems to be better to serve small amounts of protein (one to two ounces) every two to four hours rather than larger amounts every five to seven hours. (If served a steak, accept it but just eat a corner of it and sneak the remainder into a pocket or purse for future nibbling.)

The hyperactive and the Jekyll-and-Hyde, up-and-down type of person should try to plan ahead so some protein or long-term (complex) carbohydrate can be swallowed every two to four hours. This tends to nourish the brain more evenly and thus prevents the conscience from disappearing. Fatigue, depression, poor concentration, and sugar cravings result from low blood sugar levels, also.

### Breakfast

Breakfast is probably the most important meal for the school child—or anyone who needs to think in the morning. Proteins (or complex carbohydrates) are a very important part of the meal because they give up (glucose) energy slowly so the brain can work for the next two to three hours. Packaged presweetened cereal gives quick energy that is dissipated in about forty minutes. It is better to go hungry and let the blood sugar fall slowly than to eat quick carbohydrates and have a sudden fall of the blood sugar because of the overproduction of insulin.

It would be prudent to get into the child's stomach at least some food that gives up its energy slowly. Some are nauseated in the morning because they are in acidosis (check the pH of the saliva) because of something that was eaten (or not eaten) at bedtime. Breakfast consumption may hinge on the bedtime snack. A bit of protein at bedtime may keep the blood sugar from being too low in the morning. Any fruit juice with no added sugar can be laced with protein powder and given while the child is still in bed. It may make breakfast time a little more cheerful. Most protein powders are safe and an efficient way to increase the protein content of foods. They are expensive and may be dangerous if consumed to the exclusion of other foods, especially those containing potassium.

These good breakfast ideas must be prepared beforehand but will keep the ingestor in good spirits for hours. Try eating one of these every two hours and see if the body and the brain stays on an even keel until supper.

These two recipes take a little longer, but the extra energy they provide is worth the effort.

### Breakfast Crunchies

⅔ cup butter
⅔ cup or less honey
1 egg
2 Tb. brewer's yeast
1 tsp. vanilla
¾ cup whole wheat flour
½ tsp. soda
½ tsp. salt
1½ cups uncooked oats
1 cup shredded cheddar cheese
½ cup wheat germ
½ cup browned sausage, drained and
  crumbled

Cream butter, honey, egg, yeast, and vanilla until smooth.
Add flour, soda, and salt. Stir in oats, cheese, wheat germ,
and sausage. Drop by teaspoonfuls onto greased cookie
sheets. Bake at 350° for 12 to 15 minutes. Cool for a minute.
Turn onto racks to finish cooling.

Prep. time: 25 mins.  **Protein** ★★★★  **Vitamin A** ★★★
Yield: 3 dozen  **Calcium** ★★  **B vitamins** ★★★★
  **Magnesium** ★★★ **Other: phosphorus**

### Breakfast Sausage

1 lb. ground pork
1 tsp. onion powder
¼ tsp. oregano
⅛ tsp. black pepper
1 tsp. safflower oil

Mix together all ingredients except oil. Form into patties
and fry in the oil.

Prep. time: 30 minutes  **Protein** ★★★
Serves 6  **B vitamins** ★★★
  **Other: iron and phosphorus**

The following recipes for breakfast drinks might be used for those who feel they need something with protein but don't have the time. (Probably because they did not eat something worthwhile at bedtime.)


### Eggnog

2 eggs
2 cups milk
1 tsp. vanilla
2 Tb. honey (try to cut down or elimi-
     nate this)

Combine all ingredients in blender. Pour into glasses, top with nutmeg. Serve with whole wheat English muffins.

Prep. time: 10 minutes
Serves 2

Protein ★ ★ ★
Calcium ★ ★
Vitamin A ★
B vitamins ★ ★

Raw-egg consumption is not recommended on a continuing basis as they contain avidin, a protein, destroyed by heating. Avidin in large amounts interferes with the utilization of biotin. (Keep raw egg consumption down to 2 or 3 a week.)


### Orangenog

2 cups milk
3 cups unsweetened orange juice
2 eggs
2 Tb. honey (try to cut down)
Pinch of salt

Combine all ingredients in blender. Serve with whole wheat toast.

Prep. time: 12 minutes
Serves 6

Protein ★ ★ ★          B vitamins ★ ★
Calcium ★ ★          Vitamin C ★
Vitamin A ★ ★

### Breakfast Pick-up

2 bananas
1 carrot
1 stalk of celery
2 cups unsweetened apple juice
2 cups unsweetened orange juice
3 Tb. regular wheat germ
3 Tb. honey (try to use less)
1 egg

Liquefy everything in the blender. Add more orange juice to thin, if desired. Serve in glass with ice. Serve with whole wheat toast or whole wheat muffins.

| Prep. time: 15 minutes | **Protein** ★★ | **Vitamin C** ★★★ |
| Makes 4 servings | **B vitamins** ★★ | **Potassium** ★★★★ |

### High-Protein Granola

3 cups raw wheat germ
2 cups rolled oats
1 cup wheat bran
1 cup sesame seeds
½ cup soy flower oil
¼ cup oil
¼ cup barley malt extract
1 cup raisins

*Optional Additions:*

2 Tb. tortula yeast
1 cup wheat or rye flakes
2 Tb. rice bran
2 Tb. rice polishings
Pumpkin seeds
Chopped nuts
Chopped dried fruits
Coconut
Sunflower seeds

Preheat oven to 300° and toast the wheat germ and seeds lightly, turning often. Mix all ingredients except seeds and fruits in a shallow baking pan for 45 minutes, stirring every

15 minutes. Add seeds and fruit and store. A vanilla bean put in the container adds a good fragrance to the cereal. Store in cool place.

Prep. time: 1 hour
Makes 10–12 cups

Protein  ★ ★ ★
Calcium  ★ ★
Magnesium  ★ ★
B vitamin  ★ ★ ★

The following would be a good breakfast for the breakfast-haters.

### Granola Bars

6 eggs
3 cups granola cereal
1 cup currants, raisins, or dates
  (chopped)
½ cup almonds, chopped fine
½ cup sesame seeds (unhulled)
¼ cup sunflower seeds

Beat eggs in a medium-size bowl. Add remaining ingredients; mix well with a spoon. Batter will be thick. Let the mixture sit for 15 minutes while the oven is preheating to 350°. Pour mixture into well-oiled 9-inch-square pan. Press mixture into pan and smooth top. Bake for 25 to 30 minutes, or until lightly brown and firm. Remove from oven and cut into 1-by-2-inch bars while still hot. Remove from pan by loosening edges gently with a spatula. Cool. Store in an airtight container.

Prep. time: 1 hour
Yield: 3 dozen

Protein  ★ ★ ★ ★
Calcium  ★ ★ ★
Magnesium  ★ ★ ★

B vitamins  ★ ★ ★ ★
Other:  iron and
        potassium

### BREADS

Cereals, breads, and other grain products are traditional at breakfasttime. If one prepares an all-purpose dry-ingredients mix ahead of time, it might just be possible to serve your own pancakes or muffins made that morning.

### Dry Mix

> 10 cups whole wheat flour
> 5 Tb. baking powder
> 2 Tb. sea salt

Combine all ingredients; mix thoroughly and store in airtight container. Used on page 163.

Yield: 10 cups          Protein   ★ ★

                        B vitamins   ★ ★ ★

### Basic Whole Wheat Biscuits*

> 2 cups whole wheat flour
> 4 tsp. baking powder
> ¼ cup milk powder
> ½ tsp. salt
> ⅓ cup safflower oil
> ¾ cup milk

> * Thin slightly to make drop biscuits. To make pancakes or waffles, add more liquid. Omit milk and use ¾ cup yogurt. Use ¾ cup buttermilk instead of plain milk. Omit ½ cup flour and use ½ cup wheat germ. Decrease oil to ¼ cup and add ¾ cup grated cheese. Decrease oil to ¼ cup and blend ¼ cup of peanut butter into oil. Blend 3 Tb. of butter into mixture for shortcake.

Sift dry ingredients together. Blend in oil to make a mix the consistency of cornmeal. Make a hollow in the center of flour mix and pour in milk. Mix with a fork until well blended. Turn out on a floured board and knead lightly ten or fifteen times. Pat to 1-inch thickness and cut with a biscuit cutter. Bake at 550° for 12 to 15 minutes.

Prep. time: 30 minutes
Yield: 2 dozen

**Enrichments for Cereals and Breads**

Use approximately 1 part of the following enrichers to 7 parts of wheat flour. Experiment with different mixtures to vary the texture and taste.

Millet or millet flour
Flaxseed meal or seeds
Cornmeal (yellow undegerminated is best)
Sunflower seeds and flour (meal)
Soy meal, grits, or flour
Rye meal or flour
Barley meal or flour
Buckwheat flour or seeds
Cottonseed flour
Gluten flour
Potato flour
Brown rice flour or polishings
Bean flour (lima and other)
Wheat germ and bran
Sprouts (all kinds), chopped fine

**High-Protein Bread**

1 cup whole wheat flour
2 pkg. yeast
1 Tb. salt
1 cup plain yogurt
½ cup water
2 Tb. butter or margarine
1 Tb. honey
1 cup whole wheat flour
½ cup wheat germ
½ cup soy flour, sifted
6 eggs, at room temperature
8 oz. muenster cheese, grated
1½ cups whole wheat flour
3 cups unbleached flour

Mix flour, yeast, and salt in a large bowl. Warm yogurt, water, butter or margarine, and honey to lukewarm, then add to yeast mixture. Beat at medium mixer speed for 2 minutes. Add 1 cup whole wheat flour, wheat germ and soy flour, eggs and cheese. Blend, then beat at high speed for 3 minutes. Add 1½ cups whole wheat flour and enough unbleached flour to make a soft dough. Turn out onto floured surface and knead in remaining flour, kneading until smooth and elastic (8 to 10 minutes). Cover and let rest 20 minutes, then shape to fit 2 well-greased 8½-by-4½-inch loaf pans. Lightly oil the tops, cover, and refrigerate overnight. Uncover, allow to stand for 10 minutes, and bake in preheated 375° oven for 40 to 45 minutes. Cool on wire racks.

| | | |
|---|---|---|
| Prep. time: | Protein ★ ★ ★ ★ | B vitamins ★ ★ ★ |
| 40 min./overnight | Calcium ★ ★ ★ | Other: phosphorus, |
| Yields: 2 loaves | Magnesium ★ ★ ★ | iron, and |
| | Vitamin A ★ ★ | potassium |

### Easy Corn Muffins

- 1 cup yellow cornmeal (unde-germinated)
- 1 cup whole wheat flour
- 1 Tb. baking powder
- ½ tsp. soda
- ½ tsp. salt
- ¼ cup safflower oil
- 2 Tb. honey
- 3 eggs
- 1 cup plain yogurt

Stir together dry ingredients and set aside. Blend oil, honey, eggs, and yogurt with a fork. Stir into dry ingredients. Spoon into paper-lined muffin cups. Bake 20–25 minutes in preheated 375° oven.

| | | |
|---|---|---|
| Prep. time: 40 minutes | Protein ★ ★ ★ | Vitamin A ★ ★ |
| Yield: 12 muffins | Calcium ★ ★ ★ | B vitamins ★ ★ ★ |
| | Magnesium ★ ★ ★ | |

### Wheatless Crêpes

3 eggs, beaten
⅔ cup water
⅓ cup soybean flour
1 Tb. arrowroot flour
¼ tsp. salt
2 Tb. toasted unhulled sesame seeds
(optional)
Sesame oil for frying

Beat all ingredients except oil together in a medium-sized bowl. Do not overbeat; when just smooth, drop by ¼ cupfuls onto a hot griddle oiled with sesame oil. Cook until lightly browned on both sides.

Prep. time: 40 minutes          Protein   ★ ★ ★
Yield: 8                        B vitamins   ★ ★ ★

### No-Wheat Muffins

⅔ cup cornmeal
⅓ cup potato starch
2 tsp. baking powder
½ tsp. salt
½ tsp. fructose or honey (optional)
1 egg
½ cup milk or nondairy milk
1 tsp. oil

Preheat oven to 400°. Sift dry ingredients together. Beat egg slightly and add to milk. Stir into dry ingredients. Add oil and mix well. Spoon into well-greased or paper-lined muffin tins. Bake for 30 minutes.

Add ⅓ cup sunflower or sesame seeds to increase the nutritional value.

Prep. time: 45 minutes          Protein   ★ ★
Yield: 8 to 10 muffins          B vitamins   ★ ★

### Pancakes

> 2 cups all-purpose dry
>    ingredients mix (See page 159.)
> 1 egg
> ⅓ cup vegetable oil
> 2–2½ cups milk or water

Mix all ingredients thoroughly. Drop by tablespoonfuls onto a hot, lightly greased skillet. For thicker pancakes, reduce milk or water by ¼ to ½ cup.

Don't ruin the pancakes by dumping syrup, honey, or molasses on them. Use butter, nut butter, applesauce, berries, crushed pineapple, or yogurt.

Prep. time: 15 minutes     **Protein**  ★ ★ ★
Serves 4     **B vitamins**  ★ ★ ★

## SOUPS AND LEGUMES

Soup is a useful complement to sandwiches. Soup made with beans or legumes when eaten with whole-grain breads will provide the body with a virtually complete mixture of all the amino acids.

| | | |
|---|---|---|
| Barley | Beans | Peas |
| Brown rice | Black | Black-eyed |
| Buckwheat | Kidney | Chick |
| Cracked wheat | Lima | Split |
| Whole wheat | Pinto | Lentils |
|   berries | Great Northern | Soybeans |
| Bran | Red | Soy grits |
| Millet | Brown | |
| Cornmeal, whole, | Navy | |
|   yellow | Cranberry | |
| | Garbanzo | |

### Basic Bean Cookery

Sort and remove any foreign material (pebbles, discolored beans, etc.).

Soak in water (6 cups for each pound of beans) for six to eight hours or overnight. You may add 1½ tsp. salt to the rinse water, in which case none should be used in cooking.

Authorities differ on the wisdom of using or discarding the soak water for cooking the beans. Some feel beans are more digestible if cooked in fresh water; others feel you lose valuable nutrients if soaking water is discarded. However, all agree that if beans are soaked for more than twelve hours, it is best to discard the water and cook in fresh water.

Time of cooking depends on the kind of bean, its age, where it was grown, and the hardness of water in which it is cooked. A bean is done when the skin is firm and the inside soft.

In hard-water areas baking soda is often used to make beans more tender. If you use baking soda, *never* use more than ¼ tsp. in 6 cups of water. Baking soda in greater quantity will rob the beans of valuable nutrients.

A pressure cooker can cut down cooking time by more than half. Follow the directions carefully and never fill the pressure cooker more than half full of water and beans.

Cook beans before adding tomatoes, wine, or any acid. Beans accept a marinade best and fastest when they are warm.

*Storage:* Beans will keep well in the refrigerator for three to four days, and in the freezer for six months or more. If they are to be frozen, place the liquid in one container and the drained beans in another to improve the quality of any dish in which they are to be used.

Soybeans are an exception to the rule. They should be soaked three times longer than navy, pea, or pinto beans. Soybeans should be soaked for eight to twelve hours in the refrigerator and then frozen, defrosted, and cooked. This method cuts cooking time about in half.

### Basic Lentil Soup

2 lb. lentils (or 1 lb. brown rice plus
  1 lb. lentils)
2 small garlic buds, chopped
2 medium carrots, chopped
1 medium onion, chopped
2 qts. water
Pinch of salt

Wash the lentils. Put into a large kettle with water and salt. Bring to boil, then simmer until lentils are tender. Sauté the chopped vegetables in a bit of oil. Add to lentils and simmer 10 minutes. Garnish with parsley. Freeze unused portion.

*Variations*
Run final mixture through the blender and add 2 cups of cream or milk for cream of lentil soup. Sausage meat can be added. Split pea or chickpea soup can be made from the basic lentil recipe. Don't forget to add some fine herbs; basil and parsley are especially good. Try whole cloves.

Prep. time: 1½ hours

Enough for a squad of hungry farm hands (about 2 quarts)

Protein ★ ★ ★

B vitamins ★ ★ ★

With sausage, the protein content will be ★ ★ ★ ★

### Clam Chowder

4 potatoes, unpeeled and diced
1 medium onion, chopped fine
3 Tb. butter
2 cups milk
1 cup light cream
2 cans minced clams

Boil unpeeled and quartered potatoes 15 to 20 minutes or until just cooked in barely salted water. Sauté onion in butter until clear. Mash potatoes in pot and add the onion plus butter, then clams and clam juice. Add milk and cream and simmer until warm. Serve with a whole-grain bread.

Some sauté the onion in a pan with a cube of salt pork. Some dice the potatoes only.

Prep. time: 40 minutes    Protein  ★★★    B vitamins  ★★★
Serves 8                  Calcium  ★★★    Other: potassium

### Lentils and Cheese

  1 lb. lentils
  1 medium onion, diced
  2 Tb. butter
  ½ cup grated cheddar cheese, divided

Simmer lentils in enough water to cover until soft. Mash. Sauté onion in butter. Mix onion, butter, and ¼ cup cheese into lentils; season. Put into greased baking dish and cover the top with the rest of the grated cheese. Bake in 350° oven until brown. Because of the sodium in the cheese, do not salt this mixture. The potassium in the lentils helps the balance.

Prep. time: 1½ hours    Protein  ★★★★    B vitamins  ★★★
Serves: 4–6             Calcium  ★★★★    Other: potassium
                                         and iron

### Braised Chickpeas

  2 cans (15–16 oz.) garbanzo beans,
    undrained
  2 cloves garlic, chopped fine
  4 onions, chopped fine
  Salt and pepper to taste
  2 cups tomatoes, chopped, undrained
  ½ cup fresh parsley, chopped
  ¼ cup mint, chopped (optional)

Place chickpeas in heavy pot or Dutch oven, with their juice. Bring to boil. Add all other ingredients. Cook over low heat for 20 minutes. The mixture must be boiling all the time even though the heat is low. Greeks eat this during Lent. The Spanish add pieces of pork or garlic sausage.

Prep. time: 35 minutes    **Protein** ★ ★ ★    **Vitamin A** ★ ★ ★
Serves 6    **B vitamins** ★ ★ ★    **Other: iron and
    potassium**

### Seafood Ratatouille

¼ cup olive or vegetable oil
1 clove garlic, minced
2 medium onions, chopped
2 small zucchini, sliced
1 small eggplant, cubed
¾ tsp. salt
¼ tsp. pepper
¼ tsp. dried oregano
1 15-oz. can tomato sauce
1 15-oz. can mackerel or other fish,
   drained and flaked

Heat oil in large skillet. Add garlic and onion and cook until onion is tender but not brown. Layer remaining vegetables in skillet, sprinkling each layer with salt, pepper, and oregano. Add tomato sauce and cover. Cook, covered, over low heat for 15 minutes or more, until vegetables are tender. Add fish and cook until heated through.

Prep. time: 30 minutes    **Protein** ★ ★ ★ ★    **Vitamin A** ★ ★
Serves 4    **Calcium** ★ ★ ★    **B vitamins** ★ ★ ★

### Lamb and String Beans

2 lbs. lamb or lamb neck, cubed
2 Tb. oil or butter for sautéing
1 can (#2) tomatoes or 1 can tomato
    paste and 1 cup white wine or water
1 large onion, chopped
1 clove garlic, minced
½ tsp. salt
Pepper to taste
2 lbs. string beans, cut in bite-size
    pieces
1 Tb. parsley, chopped (optional)

In a large stew pot over medium heat, brown the meat, onion, and garlic with the seasoning and parsley, stirring constantly. Add tomatoes, cover, and cook until meat is almost tender. Remove the meat from the bones at this point. Add the cleaned, cut beans. Another 20 to 30 minutes of cooking would be enough. Serve hot.

Prep. time: 1½ hours   **Protein** ★ ★ ★ ★   Vitamin A  ★ ★ ★
Serves 4 to 6   **B vitamins**  ★ ★ ★   Other: iron, phosphorus, and
potassium

It is often worthwhile to serve small amounts to a child; the amount of food could be as little as two tablespoonful on a butter plate. Let the *child* finish that, then let the child ask the cook for more. Some children are immediately discouraged if they see their plate piled high with a lumberjack's fare, and they eat nothing.

## MAIN COURSES

Liver from a young calf or chicken is one of nature's best sources of vitamins and iron, but children and adults generally get nauseated at the thought of swallowing any.

This may work:

### Liver

1 lb. calf's liver
1 tsp. cinnamon
2 Tb. stone-ground flour
4 Tb. safflower oil
2 Tb. cornmeal

Put liver in freezer until slightly frozen. Cut into thin strips about 2 inches long. Mix flour and cinnamon. Dip liver into mixture. Fry in safflower oil until crisp.

For a different taste, add cornmeal to mixture and fry. Drain on paper towel. A great finger food.

Prep. time: 30 minutes
Serves 4 to 6

Protein ★ ★ ★ ★
B vitamins ★ ★ ★ ★
Vitamin A ★ ★ ★ ★
Other: iron and phosphorus

It is best to obtain the liver of a young animal, one that has not been exposed to pollutants. Some authorities insist that everyone should eat some liver weekly. If this is not possible, at least try to use desiccated liver powder in things. I've heard of some cooks who tried to sneak a teaspoon of ground liver into a pound of hamburger meat, hoping the families would not know. Kids usually know if there is liver in the house. If you cannot tolerate any kind of liver, at least fortify foods with brewer's yeast or desiccated liver powder.

### Liver Letlive

1 lb. liver
2 Tb. butter
1 pkg. onion soup mix (from health
   food store)
2 Tb. whole wheat flour
2 cups water
2 Tb. catsup (p. 266)

In skillet, brown liver in butter. Cut the liver into small pieces as it is cooking. Add soup mix and 2 Tb. flour. Slowly stir in water and catsup. Cover and simmer 10 to 20 minutes until tender, stirring occasionally. Serve over brown rice.

Prep. time: 45 minutes **Protein**  ★ ★ ★ ★       **Vitamin A**  ★ ★ ★ ★
Serves 4                      **B vitamins**  ★ ★ ★ ★ **Other:** iron

Meat loafs are usually a sure-fire way of getting many different nutrients into your child. Here are two:

### Three-Meat Loaf

      8 slices whole-grain bread
      1 cup milk or nondairy milk substi-
         tute
      2 Tb. dolomite, bone meal, or cal-
         cium lactate (optional)
      1 to 2 Tb. brewer's yeast (optional)
      1 lb. ground beef
      ½ lb. ground pork
      ½ lb. ground veal or turkey
      3 eggs
      1 medium onion, chopped
      1 Tb. salt
      1 tsp. pepper
      1 sprig fresh thyme or ¼ tsp. dried
      1 bay leaf, finely crushed
      1 Tb. chopped parsley
   Tomato juice (optional)

Soften bread in milk. Mix dolomite and yeast with bread mixture. Combine the bread mixture with all ingredients except tomato juice. Mix well by hand. Shape into an oblong loaf and place in a greased pan. When a brown crust has formed, add a small amount of tomato juice or water to the pan to be used occasionally for basting. Bake in pre-heated 325° oven for 45 minutes.

Prep. time: 1 hour      **Protein**  ★ ★ ★ ★      **Magnesium**  ★ ★ ★
Serves 8                **Calcium**  ★ ★ ★        **B vitamins**  ★ ★ ★

### Spicy Meat Loaf

1 cup Bulgar wheat (fine grind) or
   cracked wheat or Fisher's Ala
1 lb. ground round, chuck, lamb, or
   turkey
1 large onion, chopped fine (or the
   equivalent in instant onion)
1 6-oz. can tomato paste
1 tsp. curry powder
2 Tb. wheat germ
1 tsp. allspice
1 Tb. brewer's yeast
1 tsp. salt
½ tsp. pepper
Pinch of cayenne pepper
2 raw eggs
1 cup raisins or currants
½ cup chopped almonds or hulled
   sunflower seeds
1 6-oz. can tomato juice (optional)

Place Bulgar wheat in a small bowl and cover with water.
Soak until softened—about an hour. If using instant onion,
soak that at the same time with the wheat; also soak raisins
and currants. When softened, squeeze out the water with
the palms of your hands. Mix together with remaining
ingredients. Form into a loaf and place in a well-greased
loaf pan and bake in preheated 350° oven for about 45
minutes or until browned. Baste occasionally with juice, if
desired. Cool slightly before slicing.

| Prep. time: 1¼ hours | Protein ★★★★ | Vitamin A ★★ |
| Serves 6 | Magnesium ★★★ | Other: iron and |
| | B vitamins ★★★ | potassium |

## Lebanese Meat Patties (Kibbi)

*Basic mixture:*

1 cup Bulgar wheat (fine grind) or cracked
wheat or Fisher's Ala
1 lb. ground round, chuck, lamb, or turkey
1 large onion, chopped fine (or the equivalent in instant onion)
1 6-oz. can tomato paste
1 tsp. allspice
1 tsp. salt
¼ tsp. pepper
Pinch of cayenne pepper
1 to 2 eggs

*Stuffing:*

1 lb. ground beef, lamb,          Salt and pepper to taste
  or turkey                        ½ to 1 tsp. allspice
½ cup nuts or hulled              ½ to 1 tsp. curry powder
  sunflower seeds
2 onions, chopped
1 cup raisins or currants

Soak Bulgar wheat in water until softened (about 1 hour).
Check occasionally to be sure there is enough water to
cover. If using instant onion, soak that at the same time in
the same bowl. While this is soaking, make stuffing by
sautéing all stuffing ingredients in a large frying pan until
well cooked. After the hour of soaking Bulgar wheat,
squeeze the water out of it and mix in additional basic
mixture ingredients. Stuff large balls of basic mixture with
stuffing mixture. Shape like hamburgers and place on
greased baking pans or cookie sheet. Be sure that patties
are well shaped and firm by patting into shape once more,
or they will crack and fall apart. Bake in preheated 400°
oven for about 30 minutes or until done. Tops may be
brushed with butter or oil, if desired. Serve hot or at room
temperature.

Prep. time: 1½ hours  
Serves 8

Protein  ★ ★ ★ ★  
Calcium ★ ★ (add 2 or 3 Tb.  
   dolomite to mixture to increase)  
Magnesium  ★ ★ ★  B vitamins  ★ ★ ★  
Vitamin A  ★ ★      Other: iron and  
                        potassium

Very good over noodles or your child's favorite pasta.

### Wheatless Brown Sauce

¼ cup arrowroot, cornstarch, or po-  
   tato starch  
¾ cup cold beef stock  
3¼ cups hot beef stock  
½ cup tomato sauce  
1 sprig fresh thyme or ¼ tsp. dried  
½ bay leaf  
1 Tb. brewer's yeast and 1 Tb. dolo-  
   mite (optional)

Combine starch, yeast, and dolomite with cold stock. Add hot stock and blend well. Add remaining ingredients and cook over moderate heat for 25 minutes. Strain and serve.

Prep. time: 15 minutes  
Yield: 1 quart

Protein  ★ ★  
Calcium  ★ ★  
B vitamins  ★ ★

### Easy Pizza

*Crust:*  
1¼ cups whole wheat flour  
¾ cup oat flour  
1 tsp. baking powder  
½ tsp. salt  
½ cup plain yogurt  
¼ cup vegetable oil  
⅔ cup water

Stir together dry ingredients. Combine yogurt, oil, and water and add to dry ingredients. Stir and knead until dough holds together. Pat into a round pizza pan or oblong jelly roll pan. Bake in preheated 425° oven for 12 to 15 minutes.

*Topping:*

1 15-oz. can tomato sauce
2 Tb. brewer's yeast
1 Tb. Italian seasoning
1 tsp. honey
1 tsp. salt
1 tsp. dried onion

½ tsp. oregano
3 cups ground beef or sausage
2 cups grated mozzarella cheese
½ cup Parmesan cheese, grated

Combine first 7 ingredients. Brown meat and drain. Cover baked crust with the sauce, then the meat, and top with cheeses. Bake in preheated 425° oven for 10 to 15 minutes.

Prep. time: 45 minutes    **Protein**  ★ ★ ★ ★    **Magnesium**  ★ ★ ★
Yield: 1 pizza    **Calcium**  ★ ★ ★    **B vitamins**  ★ ★ ★ ★

One could substitute other meats in this one:

### Turkey Vegetable Pie

Whole-grain crust for 2-crust 9-inch
pie (page 250)

1 cup cubed carrots
1 cup cubed potatoes, skins on
1 cup chopped celery
1 cup frozen green peas
¼ cup butter or margarine
½ cup diced onion
2 Tb. soy flour

2 Tb. brewer's yeast
1½ tsp. dry mustard
½ tsp. paprika
¾ tsp. salt
¼ tsp. pepper
1½ cups chicken broth
2 cups cooked, cubed turkey

Cook carrots, potatoes, and celery in steamer until just tender. Pour boiling water over frozen peas and allow to stand 4 minutes; set vegetables aside. Melt butter and sauté onions. Blend in soy flour, yeast, and seasonings; then add broth and cook and stir until thickened. Stir vegetables and turkey into thickened broth. Turn into pie shell and top with crust, making vents for steam. Bake in preheated 375° oven for 40 minutes or until golden.

Prep. time: 1¾ hours   **Protein**  ★ ★ ★ ★   **Vitamin A**  ★ ★ ★
Serves 4 to 6          **Calcium**  ★ ★         **B vitamins**  ★ ★ ★ ★

This recipe could help make the reluctant seafood eater a seafood lover:

### Spaghetti with Shrimp

2 15-oz. cans tomato sauce
1 cup chopped onion
1 tsp. oregano
1½ tsp. basil
1 clove garlic, minced
2 Tb. honey
4 Tb. brewer's yeast
½ tsp. salt
½ tsp. pepper

¼ cup grated Romano
  cheese
½ cup grated Parmesan
  cheese
1 lb. cooked shrimp
8 oz. whole wheat
  spaghetti,
  cooked and
  drained

Combine first 10 ingredients. Simmer uncovered about 40 minutes, until thickened. Add shrimp and stir just long enough to heat. Reduce heat, add cheeses, and stir until melted. Serve over spaghetti with more cheese, if desired.

Prep. time: 1 hour   **Protein**  ★ ★ ★ ★   **B vitamins**  ★ ★ ★ ★
Serves 4 to 6        **Calcium**  ★ ★ ★       **Vitamin A**  ★ ★ ★
                     **Magnesium**  ★ ★ ★

Many of the recipes in this book are easy enough for children to prepare, and if they do the cooking, they just might eat some of it. Try to get the family or the whole neighborhood involved in this one, and the stews that follow it:

### Kids' Pot Roast

3- to 4-lb. pot roast
¼ medium lemon
2 medium onions,
    sliced thin
2 tsp. onion powder
6 small carrots, whole
⅛ tsp. garlic powder
2 tsp. safflower oil
¼ lb. mushrooms, sliced

2 medium potatoes, unpeeled
1 tsp. dry mustard
1 tsp. ground ginger
4 stalks celery with leaves,
    sliced
1 small green pepper, cut up
2 cups salt-free tomato or V-8
    juice

The night before, squeeze lemon juice over entire roast. Pierce with a fork and rub the lemon juice in. Put roast in glass container, cover tightly, and refrigerate overnight. This tenderizes the meat and is all that needs to be done to it the night before. Wash the vegetables and set out the seasonings for the next day. About 3 hours before dinner, put the roast in a Dutch oven or electric skillet. Slice vegetables. Pour tomato juice over roast. Sprinkle the seasonings on the meat. Put the onion, green pepper, and tomato on the roast and the other vegetables around it. Cover and let simmer until done. Check occasionally. Add more juice if necessary. Cook at 275° to 300° if using an electric skillet. Serve with horseradish.

Prep. time: 30 minutes one day,
            3 hours the next
Serves 6, with some meat left
over for a snack the next day.

Protein  ★ ★ ★ ★
B vitamins  ★ ★ ★
Vitamin A  ★ ★ ★
Calcium  ★ ★
Other: potassium, sodium,
    iron, and phos-
    phorus

### Hobo Stew

4 hamburger patties
4 potatoes, unpeeled
4 carrots
1 large onion, sliced

4 pats of butter
Tiny pinch of sea salt for each
    patty
4 large pieces of foil

Place foil pieces on table. One potato sliced thin for each piece of foil. Put patty on top of potato slices. Divide onion slices evenly. Slice one carrot for each pack. Add a little butter and a pinch of salt on top. Fold foil up and place packets on baking sheet. Bake in preheated 400° oven for 30 minutes or until the carrots and potatoes are done. Serve in foil.

Prep. time: 30 minutes  **Protein** ★ ★ ★ ★  **B vitamins** ★ ★ ★
Serves 4  **Vitamin A** ★ ★ ★  **Other:** iron

### Pressure Cooker Stew

    2 lbs. beef or lamb, in small cubes
    1 10-oz. pkg. frozen corn
    3 cups (or 1 28-oz. can) cooked, dried
        kidney beans (has sugar)
    2 onions, chopped
    3 medium potatoes, chopped
    1 clove garlic, minced
    ¼ cup sherry
    ¼ cup water
    Salt and pepper to taste

Combine everything in a pressure cooker or pot and cook for 20 minutes, or until tender.

Prep. time: 45 minutes  **Protein** ★ ★ ★ ★
Serves 8  **B vitamins** ★ ★ ★ ★
   **Other:** iron, phosphorus
     and potassium

Whole grain crackers or whole wheat bread would be an ideal accompaniment. I always enjoy thin cool slices of apple to nibble on if a stew is hot. A dish of unsweetened applesauce would be good with or following this.

### Joe's San Francisco Special

    2 lbs. ground chuck, lamb, or turkey
    2 Tb. oil
    2 large onions, finely chopped
    3 garlic cloves, finely minced
    ½ lb. mushrooms, sliced (optional)
    1¼ tsp. salt, or to taste
    ¼ to ½ tsp. each of pepper, oregano,
        and nutmeg
    ½ lb. fresh spinach or other greens,
        washed, well-drained and chopped
        (about 4 cups) or a 10-oz. pkg. fro-
        zen spinach, thawed, drained, and
        chopped
    6 eggs, beaten

Brown meat in oil in a large skillet. Add the onions and garlic. Continue cooking, stirring occasionally, until onions are soft. Stir in the seasonings, mushrooms, and spinach. Cook for about 5 more minutes. If using other greens, cook 15 to 20 minutes longer with cover on. Add eggs and stir over low heat until eggs begin to set. Serve immediately.

Prep. time: 45 minutes          **Protein**  ★ ★ ★ ★
Serves 4 to 6                   **B vitamins**  ★ ★ ★
                                **Calcium**  ★ ★
                                **Other: iron and vitamin A**

    This is another good example of a high-protein and high-vitamin food that can be served without the expense and the fat of animal meat.

### Mixed Bean Casserole

    2 cups (1-lb. can) cooked red beans,
        drained
    2 cups (1-lb. can) cooked lima beans,
        drained
    2 cups (1-lb. can) cooked garbanzo
        beans, drained

1 lb. lean ground beef
1 large onion, chopped
1 large clove garlic, minced
Blackstrap molasses; try to use none or
   1 tsp., not Tb.
2 tsp. dry mustard
¼ cup red wine (or ¼ cup water and 3
   Tb. vinegar)
1 can (8 oz.) tomato sauce
Salt and pepper to taste

Drain beans and save liquid in case mixture becomes too dry. Put beans in a 2½-quart casserole. Mix lightly and set aside. In large skillet cook the ground beef, onions, and garlic until the meat is lightly browned. Stir in the remaining ingredients. Add the skillet mixture to beans in casserole and mix together. Cover and bake for approximately 1 hour in preheated 325° oven.

| Prep. time: 1½ hours | Protein ★★★★ | B vitamins ★★★ |
| Serves 8 | Calcium ★★★ | Other: iron and |
| | Magnesium ★★★ | potassium |

### Refried Beans

½ lb. dried pinto beans, cooked OR
1-2 (15 oz.) cans plain pinto beans,
   drained but reserve the liquid
2 Tb. salad oil

Heat oil in a heavy skillet and add the beans. As the beans simmer, mash them with a potato mashing implement and stir. Add reserved liquid if needed. Simmer about 20 minutes stirring occasionally.

| Prep. time: 25 minutes | Protein ★★★ |
| Yield: 2–4 servings | Calcium ★★ |
| | B vitamins ★★ |

## Salads

### Lemony Bean Salad

4 cups (or 2 15-oz. cans) of lima, garbanzo, or small white beans,
  drained (which may have sugar)
  (see directions for cooking beans,
  page 164)
1 small onion, sliced into rings
2 Tb. parsley, minced finely

*Marinade:*

⅔ cup vegetable oil
¼ cup lemon juice
1 tsp. salt
½ tsp. dry mustard

About 8 hours before serving, mix the marinade ingredients
in a large bowl with a wire whisk or fork. Add the beans,
onion, and parsley and toss gently to coat well. Cover and
refrigerate 8 hours or overnight. Stir occasionally to distribute marinade.

Prep. time: 10
minutes
Serves 6

**Protein ★ ★ ★**
**Magnesium ★ ★ ★**
**Vitamin C ★ ★ (add ½ tsp.**
  **vitamin crystals to 1 Tb.**
  **water. Dissolve. Add to**
  **lemon juice.)**

**B vitamins ★ ★**

### Nutty Chicken Salad

2 cups cooked, cubed chicken
½ cup chopped celery
½ cup coarsely ground peanuts
¼ cup crushed pineapple in its own
  juice, drained
¼ cup mayonnaise
  Salt and pepper to taste

Mix all ingredients together and chill.

| Prep. time: 15 minutes | Protein ★★★★ | Vitamin C ★★★ |
| Yield: 3 cups | Calcium ★★ | Other: potassium |
| | Magnesium ★★★ | and |
| | B vitamins ★★★ | phosphorus |

### Taco Salad

Salt, pepper, and garlic powder to
taste
Italian dressing or hot sauce (optional)
1 Tb. chili powder
1 lb. hamburger, browned, drained,
    and cooled
2 cups cooked and dried pinto beans
    or 1 15-oz. can, undrained (has
    sugar) (see directions for cooking
    beans, page 164)
2 tomatoes, chopped
1 head lettuce, shredded
½ bunch green onions, chopped
½ cup hulled sunflower seeds or
    chopped almonds
1 green pepper, chopped
1 to 2 cups taco chips, chopped
2 cups cheddar cheese, shredded (op-
    tional)

Mix salt, pepper, garlic, chili powder, and Italian dressing
with hamburger. Place all other ingredients in a large salad
bowl and add the meat. Toss gently. Can also be arranged
in layers in a glass bowl, starting with lettuce on the
bottom, then the nuts, beans, onions, tomatoes, peppers,
and meat, with taco chips on top.

| Prep. time: 30 minutes | Protein ★★★★ | Vitamin A ★★ |
| Serves 6 to 8 | Calcium ★★★★ | B vitamins ★★★ |
| | Magnesium ★★★ | |

### Combination Citrus Salad

1 head romaine or leaf lettuce
3 pink grapefruit, peeled
6 navel oranges, peeled
1 cup plain yogurt
2 Tb. lemon juice
1 Tb. honey, warmed
½ tsp. vitamin C crystals
1 Tb. lemon peel, grated
¼ tsp. vanilla
Dash salt
½ cup chopped walnuts

Wash lettuce and pat dry. Tear into small pieces and place in large salad bowl. Section grapefruit and slice oranges crosswise; toss with lettuce. Dissolve vitamin C crystals in honey; combine with yogurt, lemon juice, lemon peel, vanilla, and salt. Blend until smooth. Pour over salad just before serving and toss. Sprinkle with nuts.

| Prep. time: 30 minutes | Protein ★★★ | B vitamins ★★★ |
|---|---|---|
| Serves 8 | Calcium ★★★ | Vitamin C ★★★★ |
| | Magnesium ★★★ | |

### SNACKS

### Peanut Butter and Honey Pie

1 9-inch unbaked pie shell (page 250)
4 eggs
¾ cup honey
½ cup natural-style peanut butter
¼ cup sesame butter
½ tsp. vanilla
1 cup chopped salted peanuts
½ cup unhulled sesame seeds

Beat eggs with honey. Add peanut butter, sesame butter, and vanilla and beat until creamy. Stir in peanuts and sesame seeds and turn into 9-inch unbaked pie shell. Bake in preheated 350° oven for 1 hour, until toothpick inserted in center comes out clean. Cool completely and refrigerate. Top of pie will be hard; peanuts rise to the top and form a crunchy coating.

Prep. time: 1¼ hours    **Protein** ★ ★ ★ ★    Other: potassium,
Serves 8      **Calcium** ★ ★ ★ ★      phosphorus,
     **Magnesium** ★ ★ ★      and iron
     **B vitamins** ★ ★ ★

### Blender Peanut Butter

2 cups unsalted peanuts
1 tsp. safflower oil

Put oil and a few peanuts in blender. Blend until smooth. Keep adding peanuts a few at a time until all are used.

Prep. time: 20 minutes    **Protein** ★ ★ ★ ★    **B vitamins** ★ ★ ★
Yield: ½ cup      **Calcium** ★ ★      Other: potassium
     and iron

### Peanut Butter Smoothie

1 banana
3 Tb. peanut butter, natural style
3 Tb. yogurt (plain)

Purée banana. Add peanut butter and yogurt. Blend until smooth. (Add crushed dolomite if needed.) Use for baby food or freeze for older children.

Prep. time: 10 minutes      **Protein** ★ ★ ★
Yield: Serves 2      **Calcium** ★ ★
     **Other: potassium**

### Oven-Roasted Soybeans

1 cup soybeans
¼ cup melted butter (optional)
Salt, garlic salt, or smoked salt

Soak beans overnight in salted water. Simmer in soaking water for 1½ hours. Drain well. Spread in a shallow pan and roast in a 350° oven until brown—about 30 minutes. Sprinkle with butter, if used, and salt.

Prep. time: Soaking time plus
15 minutes
Yield: 1½ cups

Protein  ★ ★ ★ ★
Vitamin A  ★ ★
Other: phosphorus and iron

### Sunny Oat Cookies

½ cup peanut butter
½ cup honey
¼ tsp. salt
1½ cups old-fashioned oats
½ cup sunflower seeds, shelled

In medium bowl, stir together peanut butter, honey, and salt until well mixed. Stir in oats and sunflower seeds. Drop by rounded teaspoonfuls onto lightly greased cookie sheet. Bake in preheated 350° oven 8 to 10 minutes until lightly browned. Cool 2 minutes. Put on wire rack to cool completely.

Prep. time: 20 minutes
Yield: 3 dozen

Protein  ★ ★ ★ ★
B vitamins  ★ ★ ★ ★

### Oatmeal Cookies

1 cup old-fashioned oats
¾ cup whole wheat flour
⅓ cup honey
½ cup chopped walnuts
½ cup shortening

¼ cup sugar
1 egg
½ tsp. salt
½ tsp. baking soda
¼ tsp. vanilla

Combine all ingredients in large bowl. Beat with mixer at medium speed, occasionally scraping sides of bowl. Drop by teaspoonfuls 1 inch apart on cookie sheet and bake 12 minutes in preheated 350° oven. Or spread mixture in a large baking pan to make bars, baking 20 minutes. Natural-style peanut butter, raisins, coconut, or grated orange peel may be added, singly or in combination.

Prep. time: 1 hour
Yield: 4 dozen cookies
or 2 dozen bars

Protein  ★ ★ ★
B vitamins  ★ ★ ★

## Main Dishes

### Ginger Beef Bok Choy

1 lb. flank steak, chuck, round, or
rump, thinly sliced (¼ inch) in 2-
by 1-inch pieces, or ask the butcher
to slice as for sukiyaki
⅓ cup fresh ginger root, peeled and
sliced vertically as thin as possible
¼ cup chicken broth or stock
1 Tb. cornstarch or more
3 to 4 Tb. soy sauce
2 Tb. oil
1 bunch bok choy stalks cut into 2-
inch strips, then again lengthwise
(save the leafy part for other dishes)

In preheated skillet or wok, place oil, sliced meat, ginger root, and soy sauce. Stir-fry rapidly for about 3 minutes at high heat. Add bok choy and stir-fry 1 or 2 minutes more. Add chicken broth combined with the cornstarch. Stir until the gravy thickens. Serve immediately with steamed brown rice.

Prep. time: 30 minutes
Serves 4 to 6

Protein  ★ ★ ★ ★
B vitamins  ★ ★ ★

Calcium  ★ ★ ★
Other: iron and
phosphorus

## Parmesan Chicken

2½ to 3 lbs. cut-up chicken
½ cup Parmesan cheese
¼ cup whole wheat flour
1 tsp. paprika
½ tsp. sea salt
Dash pepper
1 Tb. milk (optional)
1 egg, slightly beaten
¼ cup melted butter

Combine cheese, flour, and seasonings in plastic bag. Dip chicken in milk beaten with egg and coat with dry mixture. Put in baking dish and pour the butter over the chicken. Bake in preheated 350° oven for 1 hour.

Prep. time: 30 minutes  Protein ★★★★
Serves 4 to 6     Calcium ★★★
          B vitamins ★★★

## Oven-Glazed Chicken

2 frying chickens, cut up
½ cup salad oil
1 tsp. grated orange rind
½ cup orange juice
1 tsp. salt
1 tsp. dry mustard
1 tsp. paprika
¼ tsp. Tabasco sauce

Arrange chicken in single layer in large shallow pan. Brush well with mixture of oil, orange rind, juice, and seasonings. Bake in preheated 425° oven, basting often with orange mixture, for 45 minutes, or until chicken is tender and glazed a rich golden color.

Prep. time: 20 minutes  Protein ★★★★
Serves 8       B vitamins ★★★

### Chicken and Stuffing Pilaf

    2 Tb. butter
    ¼ cup chopped onion
    1 cup Bulgar wheat or soy grits
    1 cup chicken broth
    1½ cups water
    1 tsp. poultry seasoning
    ½ tsp. sage
    ½ tsp. salt
    ¼ tsp. ground black pepper
    2 cups cooked cubed chicken

Melt butter in a large skillet; sauté onions and wheat or soy grits for a few minutes until coated, stirring constantly. Add remaining ingredients, cover, and bring to a boil. Reduce heat and simmer covered for 15 minutes.

Prep. time: 25 minutes  **Protein**  ★ ★ ★ ★    **B vitamins**  ★ ★ ★
Serves 4 to 6           **Magnesium**  ★ ★ ★  **Other: phosphorous**
                        **Vitamin A**  ★ ★            **and iron**

### Chicken with Savory Rice

    1 roasting chicken, 3 to 4 lbs.
    Pepper and salt or salt substitute
    4 Tb. butter, divided
    ¼ cup minced onion
    ⅓ cup sliced fresh mushrooms
    15-oz. bottle spaghetti sauce (available
      at health food stores)
    ¼ cup sliced ripe olives
    ⅓ cup seedless raisins
    2 cups cooked brown rice
    ¾ tsp. sea salt
    ¼ tsp. oregano
    ¼ cup water

Wash chicken and rub inside with salt; sprinkle outside with salt and pepper. Melt 2 Tb. butter in a skillet, add onions and mushrooms. Sauté until tender and golden. Add spaghetti sauce and bring to a boil. Add olives and raisins and cook gently for 5 minutes. Meanwhile, add remaining 2 Tb. butter, salt, and oregano to rice and mix well. Add ⅔ cup of the spaghetti-sauce mixture to rice and mix well. Stuff chicken with rice mixture and place in shallow roasting pan. Bake 1½ hours in preheated 375° oven, basting occasionally with more melted butter. Add ¼ cup water to remaining sauce and spoon over chicken. Bake 15 minutes more.

Prep. time: 1 hour  
Serves 4

Protein  ★ ★ ★ ★  
Vitamin A  ★ ★ ★  
B vitamins  ★ ★ ★

### Chicken Tostadas

      8 6-inch corn tortillas  
      Oil for frying tortillas  
      2 to 3 whole large chicken breasts,  
         cooked and shredded  
      ½ tsp. each salt, pepper, and ground  
         cumin  
      2–3 cups refried beans  
      2–3 cups finely shredded lettuce  
      1 large avocado, seeded, peeled and  
         sliced (optional)  
      3 large tomatoes, chopped  
      1 cup green onion, finely chopped  
      1¼ cups Monterey jack cheese,  
         shredded  
      1 cup sour cream or plain yogurt  
         (optional)

In a small skillet fry tortillas one at a time in ¼ inch of hot oil for about 30 seconds on each side, or until crisp and golden brown. Drain on paper towels, then keep warm in 250° oven in a covered baking dish or in foil. Mix the chicken with the salt, pepper, and cumin. Have all other ingredients at hand. To assemble each tostada, place a warm tortilla on a serving plate. Spread with a ¼- to ½-inch layer of refried beans, spoon on chicken, then add lettuce, avocados, tomatoes, onion, cheese, and sour cream or yogurt, if used. Serve with olives and hot sauce.

Prep. time: 40 minutes   **Protein**  ★★★★     **B vitamins**  ★★★
Yield: 8                **Calcium**  ★★★       **Other: potassium**
                              **Magnesium**  ★★★


### Chili con Carne

1 lb. beef in ½-inch cubes
1 lb. ground beef
4 Tb. fat or bacon drippings
2 large onions, coarsely chopped
2 large cloves garlic, minced
4 Tb. cornstarch (plus 1 Tb. each calcium lactate and brewer's yeast [optional])
2 cups water
2 cups cooked red kidney or pinto beans*
4 Tb. chili powder
1 tsp. whole cumin or comino seeds
Salt and pepper to taste
* See directions for cooking dried beans (page 250).

Cook meat in fat in a heavy saucepan, breaking the ground beef into small particles, until meat is almost done. Add onions and garlic and cook until onions are transparent. Mix the cornstarch in a little water to make a paste and add to 2 cups water. Add this mixture to the pot and simmer at least 30 minutes. Add beans, chili powder, and cumin or comino. Add more water if necessary to make the consistency of thick soup. Bring to a simmer.

Prep. time: 1 hour     **Protein**  ★★★★     **Magnesium**  ★★
Serves 10 to 12      **Calcium**  ★★         **B vitamins**  ★★

## Cheese Enchiladas

⅓ cup vegetable oil
18 corn or whole wheat tortillas
1 10-oz. can enchilada sauce
¼ cup water
1¼ cups sour cream
1 lb. cheddar cheese, grated
1 lb. Monterey jack cheese, grated
¾ cup chopped ripe olives
1 medium onion, chopped
1 4-oz. can diced peppers, or whole
   green chilies, seeded, rinsed, and
   chopped

Combine enchilada sauce and water and heat. Using a little oil at a time, quickly dip each tortilla into hot oil, turning quickly to soften. Dip into enchilada sauce. Organize ingredients in an assembly-line order. Spread 2 Tb. sour cream down the center of each tortilla. Sprinkle both cheeses in the center generously. Sprinkle lightly with olives. Roll filled enchiladas firmly and place loose edge down in 10-by-15-by-1-inch baking pan. Pour remaining sauce over enchiladas. Top with remaining sour cream, cheeses, olives, and green pepper pieces. Bake in pre-heated 325° oven for 20 to 25 minutes until piping hot.

Three-fourths cup is a lot of olives and a lot of sodium. Guacamole salad would be a good balance; avocados have lots of potassium.

Prep. time: 1 hour         Protein    ★ ★ ★ ★
Serves 6 to 8              Calcium    ★ ★ ★ ★
                          B vitamins  ★ ★

Here are two satisfying dishes which, along with Spaghetti and Shrimp, make your child a seafood fan.

### Fish Patties

1 15-oz. can mackerel or other fish
2 to 3 Tb. parsley, finely chopped
Juice of 2 lemons
½ onion, finely chopped
2 eggs
4 Tb. wheat germ or whole wheat
  bread crumbs
1 Tb. brewer's yeast, optional
Pepper to taste
¼ to ½ cup whole wheat flour
Olive or vegetable oil

Drain fish and flake with fork. Add parsley and juice of one lemon and all remaining ingredients except for flour and oil. Form into 6 patties 2 inches in diameter. Roll them in the flour and fry in hot olive or vegetable oil for about 5 minutes, or until golden brown on both sides. Sprinkle with remaining lemon juice or serve plain or with your favorite sauce. May be served on buns as fishburgers.

Prep. time: 40 minutes          Protein    ★ ★ ★ ★
Serves 4                        Calcium    ★ ★ ★
                               B vitamins  ★ ★ ★

### Seafood Loaf

1½ cups broth or milk
  1 beaten egg
  1 tsp. onion, finely minced
  ¼ cup Bulgar wheat or soy grits, un-
    cooked
  1 7½-oz. can mackerel, tuna, or
    salmon
  1 tsp. lemon juice
Dash pepper
  1 cup frozen peas, cooked
Slivered almonds for top (optional)

Stir the first 4 ingredients together in a small bowl. Put aside. Mix together the fish and remaining ingredients in another bowl. Combine the two mixtures and pour into an oiled loaf pan. Top with almonds if desired. Bake 1 hour in preheated 350° oven.

Prep. time: 30 minutes          Protein  ★ ★ ★
Serves 3                                 Calcium  ★ ★
                                               B vitamins  ★ ★ ★

Pies, like stews, can be fun for your child to help assemble.

### Tamale-Bean Pie

1 large can (28 oz.) whole peeled to-
    matoes, undrained, or solid pack,
    mashed
2 cups (or 1 15–16 oz. can) cooked,
    dried kidney or other red beans,
    undrained, or 1 can refried beans
1 or 2 Tb. chili powder, or to taste
1 cup cornmeal
1 small can (4½ oz.) chopped black
    olives (optional)
½ cup oil or melted butter (optional)
1 large onion, chopped and sautéed
    (optional)
½ to 1 lb. ground beef, browned

Mix all ingredients together. Place in oiled casserole and bake in preheated 350° oven for approximately 60 minutes, or until done. Try to cook your own beans, as most canned beans are packed with sugar.

Prep. time: 1½ hours          Protein  ★ ★ ★ ★
Yield: 6 servings                    B vitamins  ★ ★ ★
                                              Other:  iron,
                                                          phosphorus,
                                                          and potassium

### Jiffy Tamale Pie

6 to 8 large corn tortillas, torn or cut
up into 2-inch pieces
1 lb. ground beef or turkey, or 2 cups
diced cooked chicken or light meat
of turkey
1 large onion, chopped
1 can (16 oz. drained or 12 oz. undrained) whole kernel corn, or
equal amount fresh or frozen corn
1 can (8 oz.) tomato sauce
½ cup tomato juice
1 Tb. chili, or to taste
½ lb. mushrooms, sliced (optional)
½ to ¾ cup cheddar, grated as topping
(optional)
1 Tb. oil for browning

Brown onions with meat in oil. (If the meat has already
been cooked, do not brown with the onion.) Mix all ingredients except cheese in a 2-quart casserole. Bake about 30
minutes in preheated 350° oven. Add water or more tomato
juice if the meat becomes dry. Remove from oven and put
cheese on top. Return to oven just long enough to melt the
cheese before serving.

Prep. time: 50 minutes
Serves 4 to 6

Protein  ★ ★ ★ ★
B vitamins  ★ ★ ★
Vitamin A  ★ ★ ★
Other: iron, phosphorus, po-
tassium, and calcium
(if cheese is used)

### Tofu

Tofu is soybean curd, a common protein food much
used in Oriental cooking, comparable to cottage cheese
from cow's milk. It is very digestible but very bland. It takes
on the flavor of the food with which it is cooked. The

simplest way to serve it is to mash it up, add a little soy milk to moisten, and a dash of salt. Try then to mix it with canned or fresh fruit, chopped nuts, or chives. Running some through the blender would enhance the protein value of any drink with which it would be mixed.

Protein   ★ ★ ★
Calcium   ★ ★ ★

### Tofu Surprises

2 Tb. oil
2 medium onions, diced
1 cup diced fresh mushrooms
1 cup diced tofu
2 Tb. fresh or frozen peas
2 Tb. soy sauce tamari

Heat oil and sauté onion until translucent. Add remaining ingredients and stir to heat thoroughly. Serve over brown rice.

Prep. time: 30 minutes
Serves 3

Protein   ★ ★ ★ ★
Calcium   ★ ★ ★
Other: iron

### Veal Scaloppine

1½ lbs. thinly sliced veal cutlets
4 Tb. whole wheat flour
1½ tsp. salt
¼ tsp. pepper
1 garlic clove
¾ cup butter, or less
3 tsp. salad oil
¾ lb. mushrooms
½ cup water
1 cup sherry wine

Combine flour, 1¼ tsp. salt, and pepper. In a fry pan, combine half the butter and all of the salad oil with garlic clove. Dip veal into flour mixture; brown in oil on both sides. Put veal into shallow ungreased casserole dish. Melt remaining butter, remove garlic, add mushrooms, and sauté until done. Add water, rest of salt, and wine. Scrape bottom and sides of pan. Boil and let simmer 2 minutes to blend flavors. Pour this mixture over the cutlets. Bake in covered casserole in preheated 350° oven for 30 minutes until veal is tender. Baste while baking.

Prep. time: 1 hour  
Serves 6

**Protein** ★ ★ ★ ★  
**B vitamins** ★ ★ ★  
**Vitamin A** ★ ★ ★  
**Other: potassium, iron, and phosphorus**

It would seem sensible to me to have a salad along with this. A fruit salad could act as a dessert, too. A raw vegetable salad could act as the vegetable and would add roughage, vitamin C, and some calcium. An apple or some grapes would be a neat ending to this great meal. May be a little rich for some tastes.

# Sleep 11
## Problems

Many children cannot go to sleep. Many awaken after an hour or two and cannot go back to sleep. Some sleep deeply and wet the bed. Some sleep lightly or restlessly twist and turn all night, fall out of bed, sleepwalk, or awaken screaming with a night terror. Most hyperactive children have one of these traits. There is no consistency between daytime habits and behavior and type of sleep pattern.

When the blood sugar falls through the night, the cortex may not be receptive enough to perceive that the bladder is stretched with urine. The spinal cord has no social conscience and so lets the bladder dump its load willy-nilly. The bed is wet but the child didn't do it; the bladder did. The child—the ego, the self, the cortex—was not "present." One cannot be angry at the part of the nervous system that did not know. How can one get upset with the bladder? It just knows how to fill and empty.

When ticklish, goosey, Jekyll-and-Hyde, carbohydrate-craving, deep-sleeping, bed-wetting children are fed better, many but not all stop wetting. Psychiatrists believe that many bedwetters are acting out a form of aggression (passive, urethral aggression) and are paying the mother back for real or imagined put-downs. If we can solve enuresis overnight with a diet change,* it would suggest other reasons for bedwetting. Of course, the bad self-image produced because of the wetting may have to be treated psychiatrically, but that is the purpose of this book: to correct the metabolic fault before it leads to sickness— psychological or physical.

I still wonder why some deep sleepers do not wet the bed. Paradoxically, many light sleepers have occasional "wet" nights, but I am now realizing that the fault is usually the ingestion of some food eaten only occasionally. One patient only wet on Monday, Wednesday, and Friday nights. His parents, understanding the psychogenic aspects, wondered if he hated them only intermittently until they found that he had milk and orange juice on those days and only apple juice on Tuesdays and Thursdays at school snack break. He had had terrible colic from cow's milk as a baby, asthma from cow's milk as a toddler, and now as a child the milk had turned its attention to his bladder. (He has sinus trouble if he drinks it now.)

Medical-school teaching has us believe that the person who screams out, whose heart is racing along at twice the normal rate, who has broken out in a sweat and whose pupils are widely dilated (but "the sense is shut") is having a night terror in response to some unresolved anxiety. It is certainly the end result of adrenalin secretion; this seems an inappropriate time for adrenalin to be secreted in such vast amounts. I now realize that it is usually

* For example: no dairy products. Add magnesium and a protein snack at bedtime.

a signal given off by the body to whoever will receive it that the blood sugar has dropped rapidly. When the blood sugar drops rapidly from overproduction of insulin as a result of overingestion of quick carbohydrates, the adrenal glands secrete adrenalin to help mobilize sugar from the liver to keep the sugar level at an optimum working level. The body may also assume that when the blood sugar falls rapidly some crisis is present (car or tiger coming) and that the adrenalin is also needed for flight.

Instead of asking the victim (the next day, of course) to identify the stress that could have produced such a wild night, we ask him what he ate in the six to ten hours before retiring. We are usually rewarded with a response that gives it away: "Coke and ice cream" or "bowl of dry cereal with milk and sugar." Stress or a tiger attack will certainly make the blood sugar drop, but one can handle stress more easily if the blood sugar can be maintained at a fairly consistent level with protein snacks or more slowly absorbed carbohydrates. Sleep is largely a neuro-biochemical phenomenon but is obviously affected by emotional events. One of the questions I hear most frequently is "How can I get my child to sleep through the night?" The awakening of the child is surely a neuro-biochemical event, but what he does once he is awake could be a learned or attention-getting act.

In the past, if I had already treated the child for pinworms, the only recourse I had was to knock him out with some sedative and hope he developed a "habit" of sleeping through. This rarely worked. Some of the children fell over the next day as if in a drunken stupor; it was hardly worth it.

Since I have been using a more natural, nutritional approach to the treatment of restless, wakeful children, their sleep patterns have improved. Treat the daytime problem and the nighttime disturbance ("sleep resistance" is a nice way to put it) will often clear by itself. Just supply the body with all the proper nutriments, and it will do the rest.

Inability to sleep is the brain's way of telling us "I have problems with Factor X." X may be a vitamin or mineral deficiency or not enough cortisol or seratonin or too much norepinephrine or histamine.

Sleep should be helped the most with foods containing calcium and magnesium. Tryptophan helps the brain relax and sleep and is found in most protein foods.

Tryptophan has to be given by itself (250 to 500 mg at bedtime). Tryptophan, when accompanied by other amino acids, as in a piece of meat, will not be taken into the brain in sufficient quantities to have an effect.

One doctor told me recently that he uses vitamin $B_3$ and $B_6$ for children who cannot drop off to sleep and $B_1$ for those who awaken after two to four hours of sleep. The B vitamins will usually help the brain enzymes make the necessary sleep chemicals, but some people release histamine (a stimulant) when they take a lot of Bs. If the Bs act as a stimulant, then calcium is usually needed.

One mother who had tried everything recently discovered that lecithin calmed her child, who slept and was cheerfully playing with her toys in the morning. Lecithin will provide choline, which helps the body make acetyl choline, a neurotransmitter.

Gratifying improvement is the message I get back from most parents of children with behavior and sleep problems. But even more pleasing is the change in other aspects of behavior that had not even been mentioned in the initial interview: "He stopped punching his sister." "He no longer lights fires in the wastebaskets." "She doesn't bite her nails or slam doors." "He doesn't sneeze now and can breathe through his nose."

I was helping the allergies in some, the conscience

in others; some rhythmical habits were less and, in general, these children were less sick. A nutritional approach just made their bodies work better.

### Questions and Answers

Q. My son is six years of age and has slept through the night only four times. I am surviving, but it would be nice to have a normal household. Sedatives (and we've tried them all) make him dopey or crazy. Tranquilizers work for a few nights. We've dewormed him many times. He gets up, wanders around, and crawls in with us. He goes back to sleep, but we're wide awake. If we get mad, it makes it worse. A psychologist made us feel guilty. Why me?

A. If it's any consolation, this is the most common question we get. But usually by age six children are learning to turn over and go back to sleep again. The awakening is supposed to be a biochemical defect, but the behavior afterward may be psychological. Possibly he feels rewarded for awakening.

The most effective treatment or control is the use of calcium at bedtime, especially if he has muscle cramps or craves dairy products (as if looking for calcium). About 800 to 1000 mg of calcium (as in dolomite or bone meal, or from oyster shells or gluconate) at bedtime should help him sleep all night and awaken refreshed in the morning.

Tryptophan helps some get to sleep. Magnesium and zinc may also be necessary. If the child is allergic, the nutrients that assist the adrenals might help. (Cortisone goes to the hippocampus, which helps regulate sleep.) He may be eating something that makes his blood sugar fall in the night; the adrenalin secreted at that time would awaken him. (Milk?)

Q. When I nurse my ten-month-old baby at about 9 P.M., she seems asleep, but when I try to sneak her into her crib for the night, she is wide awake and seems frightened. If I make her cry it out, she gets hysterical and may vomit everything. We're back at square one.

A. The key phrase is "seems frightened," which suggests that adrenalin is flowing. When adrenalin flows it usually means blood sugar is falling. When the sugar level falls, it has been up too high—and *that* occurred because of sugar ingestion or the intake of some food to which she is allergic. If you are giving her vitamins, it may be the sugar, color, or flavoring in them. Read the labels: certain commercial vitamins have such additives in them. Also check her diet. Would she allow another adult to put her to bed? You may be setting a pattern of nursing her to sleep.

Q. I tried the B complex vitamins on my hyperactive child, but they kept him awake. How come?

A. B vitamins have the ability to release histamine from some white blood cells, and histamine has a very stimulating effect on the nervous system. The response suggests that your child's diet needs more emphasis on calcium. Try using smaller doses and build up gradually, giving the B vitamins in the morning and the calcium at or before bedtime.

Q. My son is twelve years old and still wets the bed almost every night. On a camping trip he did not wet when sleeping in a sleeping bag on the hard ground. We now have him sleeping on the floor instead of his soft bed. I feel guilty, but he is dry.

A. Psychology, allergy, and biochemistry are all playing a part here. Psychiatrists may feel that he is angry and depressed and wets the bed to "get even" for something—what is called passive aggression. It may be true, but we believe the psychological problems develop as a result of bedwetting.

These children are usually deep sleepers because of low blood sugar following sugar consumption or foods to

which they are allergic. Food allergies don't do everything
but can do anything. Usually one knows overnight if the
offender has been discovered, although some foods may
have to be eliminated for three weeks before results are
consistent.

Try to think of what he didn't eat or drink on the trip
that he has consistently at home. (Juice on the trip and milk
at home?) Perhaps he is not sleeping so deeply on the hard
ground or floor and therefore awakens more readily when
his bladder is full. Maybe he is maturing now and his
bladder capacity is greater. When he gets back to the soft
bed, try some monetary reward, like a dollar for every dry
week. It can help. Try the Enu-Tech Co., 625 Miramontes,
Half Moon Bay, Ca. 94019. They have a system to change
sleep habits.

Let him know that you are proud of his accomplishment.

**Q. Our lovely six-month-old is fed breast milk exclusively. I eat well and nurse her when she is hungry. A pattern is developing that could lead to a problem. She is settling for a six-hour day. Eat, sing, play, and sleep four times in twenty-four hours. How do I teach her to sleep through the night like normal people?**

**A.** That's difficult to do without getting tough. She
does get rewarded for crying out, so she may have learned
that is the normal routine. One of ours did this until we put
her in a room by herself, and she slept through. I assume
our normal turnings in bed (or snoring) awakened her, and
she then awakened us. I used to sedate my wakeful patients
in the hope that they would sleep through, then eat twice as
much in the twelve daylight hours and get on a twelve
up, twelve down routine. Benadryl® and Phenergan®
worked sometimes but usually did not fix the pattern more
permanently.

In general, it is more rewarding and safer to add

calcium, magnesium, manganese, or zinc to the diet, giving each one a week to work. Some are calmed with $B_6$ or pantothenic acid. Try a juice fast for two or three days if you can—and if she is better, the problem was something you have been eating.

If all else fails, try some strained protein at bedtime. It may help her blood sugar stay up through the night better.

**Q. Our cute, active, lovable four-year-old Jason has been returned to us by the police at 5 A.M. after they found him out on the freeway in his pajamas, twice now. They said they would "take action" if we cannot control him better. He can get through any door, lock, or device short of nailing his doors and windows shut. It might be funny if it were happening to someone else.**

A. Something awakens these sensitive people, and it doesn't take much. A few dribbles of urine from a full bladder, gas going sideways, low blood sugar and adrenalin release, or low-calcium muscle cramps, a food allergy, headache, pinworms crawling out of the rectum, a nose full of phlegm from an allergy to feathers, choking from swollen floppy tonsils, a slight convulsion sending a quiver through the body is a partial list. Once up, they cannot ignore the challenge of the door or the secret of the street.

Paying attention to these inciting factors should help, but something must be done about the child's inability to disregard his environment. Calcium, $B_6$, zinc, pantothenic acid, and elimination of allergic factors should help. You may have to put a bell on him.

### Foods for Restless Kids

In general, recipes containing calcium and magnesium should be the most useful to get a child to relax and go to sleep.

One of the easiest is peanut butter (or Sesame Butter,

page 128) on a celery stalk. The long-term effect of the peanuts should prevent a fall in blood sugar. Many add calcium (oyster shell or bone meal) powder to the butter. A teaspoon of the calcium powder would be about the normal daily requirement for child or adult (1000 mg of calcium). One can call it chunky style as it's really gritty with the chalky stuff therein.

A melted or grilled cheese sandwich on whole-grain toast would supply calcium as well as protein. It should get the child down and keep him from awakening at inappropriate times.

If a child is allergic to milk and dairy products, using unhulled sesame seeds would be a good source of protein and calcium. Zorba's Delight (page 130) would be a quick way to get protein, calcium, magnesium, and the B vitamins into any insomniac. (See also Sesame Milk, page 119.)

Dr. Carl Pfeiffer of the Brain Bio Center in New Jersey has luck with vitamins C and $B_6$ and also with inositol. Vitamin C does have a calming effect (witness its use to suppress the withdrawal symptoms of drug addicts), so 500 to 5000 mg might be added to Zorba's Delight or some fruit drink.

Alfalfa and dandelion teas are two of the better-known herbal teas that provide a fair amount of calcium.

$B_6$ is almost a specific for some hyperactive children; 100 to 500 mg is quite safe. It has stopped seizures that result from low $B_6$, so it can safely induce sleep in twitchy people. And what dreams!

Inositol, anywhere from 100 to 500 mg, can calm some children at bedtime. The recipes with excellent amounts of B complex have $B_6$ and inositol as well.

Any of the recipes that have excellent sources of protein and calcium would be best offered at supper so bedtime would be a pushover. (See Spaghetti, page 133; Quiche, page 134; Whole-Grain Pocket Bread, page 139; and Animal Crackers, page 138.)

If the child falls asleep easily but awakens throughout the night—especially if she appears frightened—it suggests falling blood sugar and adrenalin release. If no sugary food has been consumed there may be an allergy, and a little detective work is needed.

This is delicious and soothing when served warm from the oven at bedtime:

### Baked Apple Surprise

Half an apple
½ cup grated cheddar cheese
¼ cup walnuts
¼ cup raisins

Slice apple thinly and place in the bottom of a 1-quart casserole. Cover with cheese, walnuts, and raisins and bake, covered, at 375 degrees for 12 minutes.

| | |
|---|---|
| Prep. time: 3 minutes | **Protein** ★★★★ |
| Yield: 1 Surprise | **Calcium** ★★★★ |
| | **Magnesium** ★★★ |

### Bedtime Cookies

1 cup raw sunflower seeds
1½ cups grated cheddar cheese
1 tsp. chives
½ tsp. salt

Process all ingredients in container of blender or food processor until dough forms a ball or holds together when squeezed. Shape into 18 to 24 balls, then press lightly with a floured glass bottom to flatten. Bake at 375 degrees for 8 to 10 minutes.

| | |
|---|---|
| Prep. time: 15 minutes | **Protein** ★★★★ |
| Yield: 18–24 cookies | **Calcium** ★★★ |
| | **Magnesium** ★★★ |

### Stuffed Celery

*For each serving:*

1 rib celery
2 Tb. pimiento cheese
1 Tb. sunflower seeds

Wash and dry celery, stuff with pimiento cheese, and top with sunflower seeds.

Prep. time: 3–5 minutes  Protein ★★★★
Yield: 1 serving  Calcium ★★★★
  Magnesium ★★★

### Fig Surprises

*For each serving:*

1 fig
1 almond
1 thin slice mozzarella cheese
  (1½″ by 4″)

Remove stem from fig and stuff with almond. Wrap cheese around and secure with a toothpick.

Prep. time: 3 minutes  Protein ★★★★
Yield: 1 Surprise  Calcium ★★★★
  Magnesium ★★★

### Snack Kabobs

*For each serving:*

1 date
2 cubes cheddar cheese
2 walnut halves

Spear a date with a toothpick; slide to center of the toothpick. On either side of the date, put a cube of cheese, then put walnut halves on each end of the toothpick.

Prep. time: 3 minutes          **Protein**  ★ ★ ★ ★
Yield: 1 kabob                 **Calcium**  ★ ★ ★ ★
                              **Magnesium**  ★ ★ ★

*Hint:* To place walnuts on the toothpicks, pierce gently, then rotate as if screwing it on the point. Do not pierce completely.

### Pineapple Sundae

1 15-oz. can unsweetened crushed
  pineapple
1 cup granola

Pour pineapple into a freezer tray early in the day. At bedtime remove from freezer, break into chunks, and blend until slushy. Divide blended pineapple into four servings and top each one with ¼ cup granola. This is especially good for the child who's used to having ice cream before bed.

Prep. time: 5 minutes          **Protein**  ★ ★ ★
Yield: 4 servings             **Calcium**  ★ ★ ★
                              **Magnesium**  ★ ★ ★

### Pizza Snacks

*For each serving:*
1 slice Pepperidge Farm Party Rye
  Bread
1 heaping Tb. browned sausage
¼ tsp. dolomite powder
1 Tb. grated mozzarella cheese

Stir dolomite powder into the sausage, top the bread with the sausage, and add the cheese. Broil for a minute or so, until cheese is bubbly.

Prep. time: 3 minutes          Protein  ★ ★ ★ ★
Yield: 1 snack                 Calcium  ★ ★ ★ ★
                               Magnesium  ★ ★
                               B vitamins  ★ ★ ★

*Hint:* I like to keep a small amount of browned sausage in the refrigerator to use in scrambled eggs, pancakes, or recipes like this. It certainly saves time to brown it in advance, but don't keep it more than three or four days.

### Popcorn Snack Mix

1 cup freshly popped corn, unsalted
2 Tb. grated cheddar cheese
2 Tb. peanuts
Parmesan cheese

Immediately after popping corn, toss with cheese and peanuts; sprinkle with Parmesan cheese.

Prep. time: 5 minutes          Protein  ★ ★ ★ ★
Yield: 1 serving               Calcium  ★ ★ ★ ★
                               Magnesium  ★ ★ ★

### Potato Stacks

1 leftover baked potato
⅜ cup shredded cheddar cheese
3 Tb. sunflower seeds
Parmesan cheese

Slice the ends of the potato off so crosswise slices will sit flat. Slice the remainder of the potato into ½-inch slices; a large potato will yield six slices. Top a slice of potato with cheddar cheese and 1 Tb. sunflower seeds. Cover with another slice, sprinkle with Parmesan cheese, and broil until bubbly.

Prep. time: 5 minutes   Protein  ★ ★ ★ ★   B vitamins  ★ ★ ★
Yield: 3 servings       Calcium  ★ ★ ★ ★   Magnesium  ★ ★ ★

### Sesame Nachos

*For each serving:*

1 nacho chip (Nachips, Doritos, or
   Tostitos are popular brands)
1 heaping Tb. grated cheddar cheese
1–1½ tsp. unhulled sesame seeds

Top the chip with cheddar cheese and sesame seeds; broil.
One child will eat 3 to 6 chips for a bedtime snack.

Prep. time: 3 minutes              **Protein**   ★ ★ ★ ★
Yield: 1 nacho (3 to 6 per serving) **Calcium**   ★ ★ ★ ★
                                   **Magnesium**  ★ ★ ★

### Banana Sandwiches

1 banana
3 Tb. natural-style peanut butter
½ tsp. dolomite powder

Stir dolomite powder into peanut butter. Peel bananas and
slice crosswise into ½-inch slices. Stuff peanut butter
between slices of banana for sandwiches.

Prep. time: 5 minutes   **Protein**  ★ ★ ★ ★   **Magnesium**  ★ ★ ★
Yield: 2 servings       **Calcium**  ★ ★ ★ ★   **B vitamins** ★ ★ ★

### Mini Tuna Burgers

1 whole wheat English muffin
⅓ cup plain tuna
Mayonnaise to spread
1–2 Tb. unhulled sesame seeds
2 Tb. grated Monterrey Jack cheese

Spread mayonnaise on muffin halves, then add tuna, sesame seeds, and cheese. Broil until cheese is bubbly.

Prep. time: 5 minutes
Yield: 1 serving (serve only ½
     muffin to younger child)

**Protein**  ★ ★ ★ ★
**Calcium**  ★ ★ ★ ★
**B vitamins**  ★ ★ ★
**Magnesium**  ★ ★ ★

Here's a great-tasting dessert drink or evening snack:

### Creamy Peanut Butter Shake

¾ cup milk
6 cubes of frozen milk (raw goat's
  milk is best, but any will work)
1 frozen banana
¼ cup natural-style peanut butter
1 Tb. protein powder (optional)
1 tsp. honey

Combine all ingredients in blender jar and process until blended thoroughly. Mixture will be very thick and creamy.

Prep. time: 5 minutes
Yield: 2 servings

**Protein**  ★ ★ ★ ★
**Calcium**  ★ ★ ★ ★
**B vitamins**  ★ ★ ★
**Magnesium**  ★ ★ ★

*Hint:* Keep peeled frozen bananas and ice-cube trays of milk in freezer, covered, ready to use.

### Mini Sprout Sandwich

*For each serving:*

1 slice Pepperidge Farm
  Party Rye Bread
1 Tb. each grated ched-
  dar and Monterrey
  Jack cheeses

½ tsp. mayonnaise
1 tsp. unhulled sesame
  seeds
Alfalfa sprouts (optional)

Top bread with mayonnaise, then add cheeses and sesame seeds. Broil until bubbly, cover with sprouts, and serve.

Prep. time: 5 minutes
Yield: 1 serving

**Protein**  ★ ★ ★ ★
**Calcium**  ★ ★ ★ ★

**Magnesium**  ★ ★ ★
**B vitamins**  ★ ★ ★

# Allergies 12

Almost everyone is allergic to some food, inhalant, or contactant to a degree. Avoidance is always the best preventative but is not always practical. Antihistamines do reduce the body's response to the sensitizing substance, but they only treat symptoms and have undesirable side effects in many people. Cortisone and similar synthetics will control allergic responses and can be life-saving, but the dangers associated with their use are so great that they are reserved for the rare and debilitating allergies and some autoimmune diseases.

Because so many victims of allergy improve with nutrition, the assumption is that we are helping the adrenal glands make their own cortisone. As proof, if vitamin C, $B_6$, and calcium are given to a victim of allergy prior to his exposure to the offending substance, he will not have an allergic response. We assume we have helped his adrenals (and other organs) produce enough cortisol (and other hormones) to interfere with the allergic reaction.

Drs. William Philpott, Marshall Mandell, Doris Rapp, and Theron Randolph have demonstrated the biochemical response of the body to ingested allergens. They chiefly affect the pancreas, but the adrenals and liver have a significant role as well. Philpott found that the blood sugar rises in most cases—which, of course, makes the pancreas secrete excess amounts of insulin, driving the blood sugar down, resulting in brain dysfunction and adrenalin secretion that produces the rapid heartbeat. It doesn't have to be sugar and quick carbohydrates that make the blood sugar bounce up and down. Philpott has discovered that some people who thought they had hypoglycemia when they ate sugar only have a hypoglycemic response when they eat cane sugar or corn syrup but not from beet sugar. This allergiclike response would help to explain normal glucose-tolerance tests in those people who thought all sugar was the villain.

It appears that blood-sugar fluctuation may not be the final traumatic event leading to various debilitating symptoms. Perhaps acidosis with its accompanying shift of potassium and sodium interferes with the normal function of brain cells (and all cells, really). Dr. Philpott recounts many cases of depression, schizophrenialike states, epilepsy, dysperception, migraine, asthma, and hives triggered by the ingestion of a favorite food.

It has also been demonstrated that when the blood sugar fluctuates from allergies or sugar ingestion, the body tends to go into acidosis. The usual energy source—glucose—is unavailable, so the body burns fat. The end products are acidic; this acidosis can have an adverse effect on the body and the brain. The saliva, intestinal juices, and the urine will become acidic to help maintain the blood at a consistent level (pH 7.4). Water is neutral (pH 7); normal saliva is slightly acidic at 6.8, but a drop of salivary pH to 5.5 to 6.0 may be associated with behavioral changes: out-of-sorts, hyperactivity, meanness, noncompliance.

A school director told me how she used this information in a practical way. The day after Easter last year she noted that about half of the students appeared restless, upset, and uncooperative. Using pH-indicator paper (from any local drug store) she found most of the children's saliva was between 5.5 and 6.5 pH. She then passed out Alka-Seltzer Gold (sodium and potassium bicarbonate, no aspirin—a teaspoon of sodium bicarbonate in a glass of water will do as well) and in twenty minutes most of them had settled down and were doing their schoolwork. Follow-up interviews indicated that most had had Easter candy for breakfast.

*Allergic-addictive syndrome* is a term that has been coined to summarize the clinical observation of this very real biochemical phenomenon. Translated into our terms: if a person loves something so much that he must have it every day, he surely has a biochemical need. When he eats a normal serving of corn (his thing), for example, his blood sugar rises and falls, his pancreas overproduces insulin and cannot manufacture the proper digestive enzymes, acidosis sets in, and potassium leaves the cells. He now craves more corn because he has found he feels better if he has it. Relief is only temporary, since the rise in blood sugar lasts only a few minutes to an hour or so before he is back on the downhill path again. Much like alcoholism. (Ninety percent of alcoholics have hypoglycemia.)

Dr. Philpott has discovered that the acid fluid of the duodenum and small bowel prevents proteolytic digestive enzymes from becoming fully active. The foods are not digested properly and will ferment or become irritating chemical peptides that act as symptom-producing allergens. It is postulated that some peptides act as morphine-like substances, thus the victim re-eats the food that makes him feel good. He must also have it frequently because he begins to feel terrible when it is not consumed.

We all have our favorite foods, and in that fact lies the method of analyzing one's own biochemical idiosyncracies. If you love something, it is probably bad for you. (Craving water when thirsty is not the same thing.) If you must have coffee several times a day, your body is telling you that you have hypoglycemia because the caffein in the coffee helps get sugar out of the liver. Or the coffee itself causes the sugar fluctuations that cause the coffee cravings.

I've been there myself. Just about 10 P.M., January 13, 1979, I realized I was drinking coffee out of the pot. I figured "There is something wrong with someone who must drink coffee out of the pot." So I quit, but not without a few clues for ten days or so that I had been hooked: terrible withdrawal headaches, surliness, glumpiness, poutiness, restlessness, even insomnia. My lifelong love affair with coffee was trying to tell me that I had (have?) a biochemical fault or two. It meant I was hypoglycemic but also, if I had really analyzed my addiction—especially drinking several cups at bedtime to promote sleep—love of stimulants to calm me must be the clue that I am hyperactive. Now finally at my advanced age I know what to do for my genetic torque. (This practical and fairly simple method of determining one's own bodily needs and acting upon the information is called folk medicine and was the best preventative we had before we began to rely on the medical profession. The latter, as a group, became so busy dealing with the diseases that they had no time to analyze the clues that were the harbingers of those diseases. Apparently we cannot let something so important as sickness be left *entirely* to the doctors.)

Assuming that most allergies become manifest because the exhausted adrenals are not producing cortisol, one should consume those foods that would compensate. A piece of fresh, raw adrenal gland would be ideal but impractical. A number of companies now market adrenal glands dried and pressed into tablets. These extracts would provide the body with the proper amounts or nutriments for that gland.

Vitamin C is stored in the adrenals and is probably the most important nutrient for the allergic person. (Primitive Northern Canadian Indians eat raw fresh adrenal glands as their chief source of vitamin C.)

Pantothenic acid is in almost all foods and is a precursor of cortisol. Big doses (500 to 1000 mg) several times a day may be necessary along with C to control allergic symptoms.

Vitamin $B_6$-bearing foods help. Calcium, vitamin A, and zinc are important to make the adrenals function better. Allergic symptoms create a stress that exhausts the adrenals, which make the allergy worse. Stress leads to stress. If stress can be anticipated, the above nutrients or foods containing them should be consumed before the stressful event.

People who eat sugar, boxed cereals, and white-flour products are more likely to develop allergies because these foods are devoid of B vitamins. The body must deplete its meager stores to digest these empty foods, since no food can be metabolized without sufficient B complex. The blood-sugar fluctuation that results from sugar ingestion will stimulate the adrenal glands to secrete cortisol. This is used for stress and then might be in short supply when needed. If the body is depleted of cortisol, an allergy could appear.

The most common food allergies are those to milk, wheat, eggs, corn, citrus, and nuts.

Most pediatricians know of the tension-fatigue syndrome so common in children. Any food can cause this, but milk and wheat are probably the most common ones. The victim is usually pale and has dark gray or purple circles under his eyes. He often has a nose full of clear or green

phlegm that seems to hang down the back of his nasophar-
ynx; he is constantly zonking, sniffing, snorting, or clearing
his throat. He acts as if a handful of rubber bands is hanging
down his throat. It usually takes about two to three weeks
of stopping the offending food before the symptoms re-
solve. Consult your doctor in the interim.

Many children outgrow their allergies. Shots and
oral drops help to desensitize; eliminating the allergen
relieves it some; avoiding emotional stress and eating only
nutritious foods all help. The following vitamins and minerals all help the adrenals make cortisol:

*Vitamin C.* The amount does not depend on weight
but on severity of symptoms. Increase the dose daily by 500
mg until the stools loosen some, then cut back a little.
Usually allergic children end up at about 2000 to 8000 mg.
If stress or symptoms appear, this daily dose is then given
hourly until the symptoms abate and the dose is cut
accordingly. A time-release capsule at bedtime may control
the early-morning sneeze.

*Pantothenic acid.* This is in almost all foods, but
allergic people need more to shore up the adrenals. It
works well with vitamin C but is very sour. Somewhere
between 500 and 2000 mg a day should help. (See recipes
with ★ ★ ★ ★ B vitamins.)

*Vitamin B₆.* Pyridoxine helps many enzyme functions in the body and seems to help the adrenals do their
job. One hundred to 300 mg a day is about right.

*Calcium.* This helps counteract the stimulating effects of histamine. We all need about 1000 mg a day;
hyperactive children should have theirs at intervals
throughout the day. Most people take it at night because of
its calming effect. Vitamin C promotes its absorption. (See
high-calcium recipes in Chapter 9.)

*Vitamin A.* If an allergic child had small bumps on
the backs of the arms and thighs and warts are present,

vitamin A should be helpful in allergy control. Probably at least 10,000 units to 25,000 units would be helpful. Some need bigger doses for short periods of time to get the control launched, then they back off to a maintenance dose.

*Zinc.* This mineral seems to be involved in a great number of enzyme functions related to skin, membranes, and the intestines. Acne victims and those with white spots in the nails would find that 30 to 60 mg of zinc a day will help their allergies also. Look for recipes with nuts, seeds, whole grains, meat, fish, egg yolk, fowl, and brewer's yeast. Any processed food is usually devoid of zinc.

It takes too long to try to solve the nutritional deficiencies of the adrenals with foods alone. Usually pills, powders, or shots of the above vitamins and minerals have to be used to get the victim out of his nutritional hole. Then the foods that have higher amounts of these things might just continue the improvement.

Nutrition-oriented doctors, such as William Philpott, Marshall Mandell, Theron Randolph, Billy Crook, and Doris Rapp, recommend that we all aim for the four-day rotation diet. Basically, do not eat any food more frequently than once every four days, especially those with the more common allergens such as dairy products, wheat, eggs, corn, potatoes, and citrus.

Many allergists do "provocative" testing, dropping extracts of various foods just under the tongue. A sensitive patient will develop a cough, a rash, a runny nose, a headache, or just about any symptom.

After complete testing, extracts of offending foods are put into a dropper bottle in the proper proportions, and parents administer this daily under the tongue and effectively control the symptoms. This is related to homeopathy.

Dr. Philpott noted that if a patient was having a symptom from a food, an extract of that food (small amount) administered under the tongue will usually stop the symptom immediately.

The pulse test has proved helpful in pinpointing allergens. The basic principle is that adrenalin is released in most people when the blood sugar falls. The adrenalin, of course, makes the pulse rate rise. Usually a twenty-to-thirty-beats-per-minute rise is needed to be certain of a definite relationship. For example, the basic resting pulse is sixty to sixty-five beats per minute. The child eats two tablespoons of corn; pulse in half an hour is ninety beats per minute. Discontinue corn.

Reading labels on packages and cans is a must. The food-processing companies are clever; they use many types of sweeteners, so no one kind is obvious. Adding all the corn sweeteners, dextrose, sucrose, honey, fructose together, one finds sugar becomes the number-one ingredient.

The Chemical Cuisine chart from the Center for Science in the Public Interest lists some common additives:

SAFE:    Ascorbic acid, carotene, calcium propinate, carageenan, casein, citric acid, EDTA, glycerin, vegetable gums, hydrolyzed vegetable protein, lactic acid, lactose, mono- and diglycerides, polysorbate, sodium benzoate, sorbitol. Many of these are naturally components of foods.

CAUTION:    May be unsafe or is used in food we eat too much of, such as soft drinks and beer, fats and fat-containing foods, cereals and desserts: BHA, MSG, phosphoric acid, phosphates, propyl gallate, sulfur dioxide, sodium bisulfite.

AVOID:    Either unsafe or inadequately tested: artificial colors, BHT, brominated vegetable oil, caffeine, quinine, saccharin, sodium nitrite, and nitrate. In this group, sugar and salt are listed, not because they pose any hazard *if one does not overuse* but because many of us do consume too much for good health.

Some people may be allergic to the water they drink. Allergic reactions can range from headaches, sore throats, runny noses, and diarrhea to depression, arthritis, and seizures. Chlorine, fluorides, and other unidentified agents in the water can cause the problems. Distilling the water gets rid of some of them. Bottled water isn't always the answer either, since its quality varies—depending on its origin, its treatment, and its distribution. Frequently, untreated spring water, with its bacteria and viruses, is bottled. Often bottled water is merely tap water run through a filter, which removes the taste and odor of chlorine but does not affect impurities.

Water bottled in plastic contains contaminants leached out from the plastic container. Water bottled in glass is a rarity, especially water that has been tested frequently for bacteria and viruses. Although the Food and Drug Administration has standards for bottled water, it cannot test each and every bottle.

If you want to filter your own water with an attachment to your kitchen sink, use a filter with activated granular carbon. This will filter out the organic matter rather than just remove solids so the water will look clear. Another good suggestion is to add a "polishing filter" that will remove any carbon as well as other particles in the water.

A final piece of advice is to rotate your water sources periodically, just as you do your food, to avoid becoming allergic to any one kind.

### Help for the child allergic to milk

Read the labels on food products carefully to avoid the hidden milk in them. Milk *may* be found in the following foods:

| | | |
|---|---|---|
| Bavarian cream | crêpes | pancakes |
| biscuits | curd | pie crust |
| bisques | custards | popcorn |
| blancmange | doughnuts | popovers |
| boiled salad | eggs, scrambled and | puddings |
| dressings | escalloped dishes | quiches |
| bologna | flour mixes | rarebits |
| bread | fondues | salad dressings |
| buns | fritters | sausages |
| butter | gravies | sherbets |
| cakes | hamburgers | soda crackers |
| candies | hot dogs | soufflés |
| cheeses | Junket | soups |
| chocolate or | mashed potatoes | spumoni |
| cocoa drinks | meat loaf | waffles |
| chowders | muffins | whey |
| cookies | omelets | white sauce |
| cream | oleomargarine | Zweibach |
| creamed foods | Ovaltine | |

**A Simple Test for Milk
and Other Food Allergies**

Cut milk completely out of your child's diet for four and a half days. Read the labels on everything he ingests to be sure milk isn't bootlegged into him through canned soups, bread, and so on. At noon on the fifth day, have him drink one large (8-oz.) glass of milk. Watch for a reaction during the next hour. If no reaction, give an additional one-half glass of milk an hour after the first try. Watch for a reaction to that during the remainder of the day and for the next few days (with no additional milk or milk products given, of course). Ideally you should have him off milk and watch for three weeks after, since that is how long it takes to get it out of his system.

Your child may react to the milk and not to cheese, so repeat the test (after three weeks), giving no milk or milk products for the required four and a half days. Give cheese on the fifth day at lunch as you did in the milk test, but use a good-sized serving of cheese. Be sure to use uncolored cheese such as cottage cheese, Monterey jack, mozzarella, or white cheddar since you want to test the cheese and not the food coloring. Some people need to stay off a food for twenty-one days to get rid of the symptoms, especially if they have the tension-fatigue syndrome.

### Egg Allergies?

Tofu, a soybean product, can be used as a substitute for eggs in certain recipes. For example, two ounces of tofu can be used for each egg substituted in pancake batter. An excellent cookbook for this food is *The Tofu Cookbook* by Cathy Bauer and Juel Anderson (Rodale Press, 1979).

Read labels carefully to determine if eggs are used in the product. Be aware that they may be present in some of the foods listed below:

| | |
|---|---|
| bakery products | meatballs |
| breaded foods | meatloaf |
| breads | pancakes |
| cake mixes | pasta |
| custards | puddings |
| ice cream | salad dressings |
| ices | sauces (hollandaise, Béchamel, etc.) |
| icing and frosting mixes | |
| malted milk and chocolate drinks | waffles |
| mayonnaise | wines (believe it or not, many wines are cleared with egg whites) |

### Questions and Answers

**Q. I was sick during the pregnancy with Beth. I had nausea and vomiting, a kidney infection, intestinal flu, then some spotty bleeding, and only gained seventeen pounds.**

Beth has hay fever, an itchy skin rash, and cannot drink milk or eat peanuts or she gets diarrhea. Is there a connection?

A. Almost every allergic child I see has come from a woman who had stress or a sickness or an accident during the pregnancy. The stress may not seem so great or obvious, but she perceived it as stressful, such as a pregnancy that occurred within two years of the last pregnancy. Stress affects to variable degrees the adrenal glands; cortisol levels will rise; then, if nutrition is not optimal, the levels fall, and in the absence of enough cortisol, allergies appear.

The baby shares the mother's ecological environment. If her adrenals go, so will the baby's. And frequently the mother is so exhausted and depressed after the debilitating nine months that she is not up to nursing—the one thing that might have attenuated the allergies. The sicker the mother or the more traumatic the delivery, the more likely is the baby to become allergic. The severity is also dependent on the incidence of allergies in the family.

Q. If I had a milk allergy as a child, could I avoid a similar problem with my child if I drink no milk during the pregnancy and while I'm nursing? Will that prevent a milk allergy?

A. Maybe. Anecdotal evidence seems to indicate that if the pregnant woman consumes no dairy products, her child may be less allergic to milk. But if one aspect of the allergy susceptibility is the state of the adrenals, it makes most sense to increase the supplements that support those glands. Vitamin C should be increased until the stools become a little loose (1000 to 10,000 mg a day). Pantothenic acid in doses of 500 to 5000 mg a day; $B_6$, 50 to 100 mg; calcium (in bone meal or dolomite), 1000 mg a day (doubled during pregnancy if dairy products not being consumed); vitamin A, 10,000 units to 20,000 units a day; and zinc (30 mg is about right) all help the adrenals work better. I would recommend this to all pregnant women who have allergies in the hope that the child would be less allergic. It would be advisable for women who are sick or stressed in some way to follow the same program. I am assuming that they are following the no-sugar, no-additives, and nibbling-six-times-a-day diet and are planning to nurse their children. Preventive methods are easier than treatment once the problem is established.

**Q. I nursed the baby exclusively for six months. Then everyone said I should quit. He got a cold and an ear infection within three weeks. He has a new rash on his bottom from the cow's milk, and he is fussy, gassy, and wakeful. I want to stop the cow's milk. What should I do?**

A. Raw goat's milk seems to be the safest. Soybean milks often use sucrose or corn syrup as a sweetener. Try to find a milk that uses lactose. Lamb and amino-acid milks work well. Some babies become allergic to all these and the milks must be rotated (cow's in the morning, soy at noon, goat's in the afternoon, and lamb milk in the evening) so they don't get a lot of any one. Boiling may help.

The basic problem may be the adrenals or the baby's immune system. It takes time, but you can get most of the essentials down the baby and build up the adrenals with your own formulation as an occasional alternate; for a fifteen-to-twenty-pound six-month-old, about a quart of fluid (water) is about right for one day. Dump ten to twelve teaspoonfuls of a good protein (strained veal or lamb) into the water and for the calcium add a half-teaspoonful of dolomite powder and a half-teaspoonful of bone-meal powder. Add the contents of a B complex capsule with 50 mg of each of the Bs. Add 250 mg of vitamin C powder, 500 units of vitamin D, and 10,000 units of vitamin A. Lactose powder would be the best carbohydrate to use; ten to twelve teaspoonfuls are about right for a quart. There is no fat in this except what is in the meat, so it is not a perfect food and would only be a stopgap measure. The formula must be shaken constantly as the solids settle to the bottom.

**Q. My child is fair with pale skin, blue eyes, and blond hair. He has blue circles under his eyes and snorts a lot. He has occasional head- and stomachaches. What is going on?**

A. That is called tension-fatigue syndrome. It is caused by a food allergy, usually milk. It takes about three weeks to get the food (egg, wheat, corn, or whatever) out of the system—usually the food the child loves. I have noticed that some children who seem to be allergic to milk have no trouble on raw certified milk. (Try to find it.) Apparently the homogenization or pasteurization or addition of irradiated ergosterol makes the milk allergenic to some children. (See no milk recipes.)

Many children have had their tonsils and adenoids removed since it was assumed that the noisy breathing, the open mouth, and the frequent superimposed infections were results of obstructive tissue. It is always embarrassing to find that the operation solved nothing at best and frequently set up a susceptibility to lung infection and asthma.

After a period of time off the milk, you may find he can drink some without the symptoms recurring. It is hard to get enough calcium (about 1000 mg a day) when off milk, so add dolomite, bone meal, or some calcium-magnesium-phosphorus-vitamin-D mixture from the health food store.

**Q. My child did have a milk allergy as a baby—colic, phlegm, diarrhea, rashes, wheezing—but seems to have outgrown it. He loves, even craves, milk now. He has insomnia and occasional muscle cramps. He seems a little hyperactive, the teacher says.**

A. He may still be allergic to milk. Perhaps his intestines are rejecting the milk—or the calcium part of it—because of the allergy. He swallows the milk because his body is begging for calcium; usually, the greater the craving, the lower the calcium level.

You must try to stop the milk and get some calcium into him, especially at bedtime, for the insomnia. You also should do something to build up his adrenals. One allergy can lead to another. A future stress might allow him to become allergic to animals or house dust.

Allergic people have very little margin of safety. An allergy to one thing, even just a sneeze or two when the lawn is mowed, is the clue that the body is compromised. The body is telling its owner "Help! I'm allergic." If some preventive measures are taken (for example, avoiding allergens, sugar, junk, and milk—if there was a past history of allergy to it) and attempts made to build up the adrenal glands, maybe one can avoid more serious allergic problems such as asthma or allergic swellings or shock.

**Q. OK, I had stress during the pregnancy, a tough delivery, and was too exhausted to nurse my son. He now has a cold and cough when he drinks milk or pets the cat. He screams with gas and diarrhea if he eats wheat, and eggs will break him out and swell up his lips. He hates all vegetables and so exists on hamburger patties, rice, apple juice, bananas, and Cheerios. How do I improve his diet and his allergies? He is two years old and whines a lot.**

A. It's too bad that your obstetrician did not do a little prevention by urging a stress formula upon you. A vitamin B complex shot every week or two might have helped your body handle the stress, physical or emotional. The La Leche League should have been called to act as your rooting section.

Actually the diet he is on is not bad as a compromise. Normal two-year-olds eat very little, whine a lot, and practice noncompliance. The obvious things he is missing are calcium, magnesium, vitamin A, and roughage.

Try the recipes that incorporate calcium (1000 mg

per day) and minerals. Vitamin C is usually low in allergic people, so adding the powder (calcium ascorbate is less sour) to the apple juice until his stools are sloppy (then reduce the dose to the subdiarrhea level) should help the allergy—500 mg on up to 5000 mg per day. Vitamin A drops (as in cod-liver oil) up to 20,000 units a day also help allergies. Could you grind up a little liver and mix it with the beef? Not too much to start or he will never eat another patty. The B complex is the tough part to get down unless he likes the flavor of dirt.

**Q. My eight-year-old girl is asthmatic. If the weather changes or she gets a cold or she overexerts, she will have an attack. We have her on a lot of drugs. They help but also make her hyper and crabby. We are just controlling symptoms. I would like to make her body well. We have allergies in the family. She had a milk allergy, her tonsils have been removed, and some attacks require anti-biotics.**

A. A common question. I assume you have her off milk. Milk, wheat, grass, pets, and house dust could all be building up so she is like a loaded gun. The trigger that sets off the attack is a weather change or other stress. Unload the gun by making your home as dust-free as possible, have only outdoor pets and electric heat in her room. No feathers, no wool, no kapok or down comforters, and so on. Allergy testing may help you pinpoint the inhalant offenders. Newer blood tests can give clues about foods. (Skin tests are generally worthless for foods.) Be sure the vitamins she takes are free of food coloring, sugar, and starch—they are potential allergens. Most natural food stores sell vitamins without these additives.

Calcium can have a calming effect on the bronchial-tube muscles that go into spasm during asthma. It and magnesium can also have a tranquilizing effect on the part of the brain that perceives stress. Use the maximum vitamin C dose her bowels can tolerate; then, when it looks like she is going to have an attack, or the weather changes or a stress can be anticipated, give the daily dose hourly. Usually overnight the attack can be aborted.

If the wheezing seems to be of an infectious nature, a course of dead-bacteria vaccine shots will often improve the immune system against the usual bacteria that cause bronchitis.

The fact that an injection of cortisone will usually stop most all allergic conditions (hay fever, asthma, eczema, hives, bee stings, and the like) suggests that the victim's adrenals are not producing enough cortisol. We now know what to give to help, but it is slow. We recommend that the patient get the routine allergic workup, but at the same time assume that the child would not be allergic if the adrenals were working properly.

The recipes that follow are rich in vitamins A and C, two helpful antiallergy nutrients. Try them. Don't be afraid to add some extra vitamin C to most of these if you have an allergic child or a family susceptible to infections. Vitamin C crystals or sodium ascorbate powder is the cheapest and usually the purest form. One teaspoon supplies about 4000 mg of vitamin C. One-fourth to 1 teaspoon of the powder is dissolved first in a tablespoon of warm water and then added to the drink or the salad or whatever.

Other sources of fair amounts of vitamin C: alfalfa, burdock, boneset, catnip, cayenne, chickweed, dandelion, garlic, hawthorn berry, horseradish, kelp, papaya, parsley, plantain, red raspberry leaf, rose hips, strawberry leaf, and watercress.

## Recipes with High Amounts of Vitamin A

Vitamin A-containing foods should be encouraged in those who use their eyes a lot or complain of eyestrain or visual difficulties in dim light or rough skin on the upper arms and thighs. Vitamin A may help control infection when vitamin C is not helpful. It helps those with allergies.

Great sources are liver (which lots of kids or parents won't eat), carrots, sweet potatoes, dried apricots, and green peppers. Greens, giblets, winter squash, canned or cooked pumpkin, spinach, butter, broccoli, and peaches are also excellent sources of carotene, a vitamin A precursor.

Good sources of vitamin A include alfalfa, burdock, cayenne, dandelion, garlic, kelp, papaya, parsley, red raspberry leaf, red clover, and yellow dock.

## Snacks and Desserts

### Apricot Butter

1 lb. dried apricots
Water or fruit juice (apple, orange, or pineapple) to cover
Pinch of cinnamon

Put apricots in a medium-sized saucepan. Pour in just enough juice or water to cover. Bring to a boil, then turn down heat and simmer covered for about 10 minutes. Remove from heat and cool slightly. Add cinnamon. Put about 2 cups of the mixture in a blender, put on lid securely, and blend at low speed until the mixture is desired consistency. Add more liquid for a thinner butter. Pour into a jar with a tight-fitting lid. Continue with remaining apricots until all are blended. Store in refrigerator and use on breads, waffles, pancakes, for sandwiches, and in beverages.

Prep. time: 45 minutes
Yield: 3 cups

Vitamin A  ★ ★ ★ ★
Other: potassium,
         phosphorus,
         and iron

### Dried Fruit Jam

1 lb. dried apricots, figs, currants,
    peaches, prunes, or a combination
    to total 1 lb.
2 cups liquid mint tea or Constant
    Comment tea
1 cup apple cider
¼ tsp. salt
2 Tb. arrowroot
Grated rind of one orange or lemon
Cinnamon, nutmeg, or other preferred spice

Soak dried fruit overnight in tea and cider. Add salt and
simmer in a covered pan for 1 hour. Cool. Purée fruit in a
blender or food mill. Mix arrowroot thoroughly in purée.
Add rind and spice. Simmer for about 10 minutes, stirring
to prevent sticking. Chopped nuts may be added when jam
is cooled. Will keep for about a week in refrigerator.

Prep. time: 1½ hours          Vitamin A   ★ ★ ★ ★
Yield: about a pint               (with apricots or peaches)
                              Other: potassium, iron, and
                                  phosphorus

### Carrot Smoothie

1 banana
2 cooked carrots
3 Tb. plain yogurt (up to ½ c)

Purée bananas and cooked carrots in the blender. Add
yogurt. Blend. (This will make a couple of meals of baby
food.)

Prep. time: 5 minutes         Calcium   ★ ★
Yield: 1 cup                  Vitamin A   ★ ★ ★ ★
                              Other: potassium

## Pumpkin Cookies

½ cup salt-free margarine or butter
1 tsp. vanilla
1 6-oz. can frozen unsweetened
   pineapple concentrate, thawed
2 eggs
1½ cups cooked pumpkin
1 tsp. cinnamon
4½ tsp. baking powder
½ tsp. nutmeg
2½ cups stone-ground wheat flour
1 cup raisins
1 cup salt-free nuts, chopped

Mix margarine, vanilla, and pineapple concentrate. Add eggs and pumpkin and stir. Mix remaining ingredients (except raisins and nuts) and stir into pumpkin mixture. Add raisins and nuts and stir well. Cover a cookie sheet with foil; grease surface of foil. Drop by spoonfuls onto cookie sheet. Bake in preheated 375° oven for about 15 minutes.

Prep. time: 45 minutes    **Protein**  ★ ★ ★    **B vitamins**  ★ ★ ★
Yield: 3 dozen            **Magnesium**  ★ ★   **Vitamin A**  ★ ★ ★ ★

## Jack-o'-Lantern Pie

1½ cups cooked pumpkin
¾ cup honey
   Pinch soda
½ tsp. salt
1 tsp. cinnamon
½ tsp. ginger
¼ tsp. nutmeg
½ tsp. cloves
1 tsp. vanilla
4 beaten eggs
1½ cups plain yogurt
¼ cup melted butter
1 10-inch pie shell, unbaked

Mix pumpkin, honey, soda, and seasonings; beat well. Add eggs, yogurt, and butter and beat until thoroughly mixed. Pour into unbaked pie shell and bake in preheated 375° oven for 1 hour, or until knife inserted in center comes out clean. The honey will produce a shiny appearance on the top of the pie; be careful not to overbake because it doesn't look done.

Prep. time: 1¼ hours  Protein ★ ★
Serves 8     Calcium ★ ★
        Vitamin A ★ ★ ★ ★

### Avocado Salad

7 avocados, peeled and pitted, medium-sized
4 tomatoes
8 green onions
3 Tb. fresh lemon juice
Salt and pepper to taste

Dice avocados and tomatoes and combine in a bowl. Chop and add green onion, then lemon juice, salt, and pepper. Add more lemon juice if desired.

Prep. time:  Magnesium ★ ★ ★  Other: potassium and
30 minutes  Vitamin A ★ ★ ★    phosphorus
Serves 12  Vitamin C ★ ★ ★

### Broccoli and Cauliflower Salad

1 small bunch fresh broccoli
1 small head cauliflower
1 cup French dressing (page 266)

Wash broccoli and cauliflower. Separate into flowerets, using just enough stem to hold the flower on. Combine in large bowl; add dressing, toss, and chill.

Prep. time: 10 minutes Protein ★ ★  Vitamin C ★ ★ ★
Serves 4     Calcium ★ ★ ★  Other: potassium
        Vitamin A ★ ★ ★

### Fresh Fruit Food

5 ripe bananas
3 ripe apricots

Mash bananas. Cut up apricots and purée in blender.
Combine mixtures and mix well. Pour into freezer tray and
freeze until edges begin to harden. Then spoon mixture
into bowl and beat with electric mixer until light and fluffy.
Refrigerate until served.

Prep. time: 20 minutes         Vitamin A  ★ ★ ★ ★
Yield: 2½ cups                 Other: potassium

### Lebanese Garden Salad (Tabooli)

¾ cup Bulgar wheat, cracked wheat,
   or Ala
2 bunches parsley, stemmed and
   finely chopped
3 tomatoes, chopped
1 bunch green onions, chopped
1 cucumber, chopped (optional)
Juice of 3 lemons
½ cup olive or vegetable oil
Salt and pepper to taste
Lettuce or romaine leaves
Mint sprig, chopped (optional)
Black olives

Soak the wheat in water for at least half an hour. Drain and
squeeze out water with hands. Mix all but last 3 ingredients
in a large salad bowl. Serve on lettuce leaves. Garnish with
mint and olives.

Prep. time: ½ hour          Protein  ★ ★ ★
Serves 5 or 6               Vitamin A  ★ ★ ★
                           B vitamins  ★ ★ ★

### Oriental Green Salad

1 bunch bok choy leaves, torn or
  shredded
½ cup almonds, filberts, or Brazil nuts
½ cup raisins or currants

Dressing
¼ cup vegetable oil
1 Tb. honey
2 tsp. soy sauce, or to taste
½ tsp. paprika (optional)

Combine the dressing ingredients in a jar with a tight-fitting lid. Shake well and refrigerate. Combine first 3 ingredients and toss to mix. Just before serving, shake the dressing and pour over salad, tossing to coat greens.

Prep. time: 10 minutes     **Protein**  ★ ★          **Vitamin C**  ★ ★ ★
Serves 6                   **Vitamin A**  ★ ★ ★     **Other: potassium**


## VEGETABLE AND SIDE DISHES

### Savory Stir-Fried Broccoli

¼ cup safflower oil
¼ cup chopped green onions with
  tops
1½ tsp. fresh minced garlic
  2 cups fresh broccoli, cut in 4-inch
  pieces
¼ cup water
¼ tsp. seasoning

Heat oil in skillet over medium-high heat; sauté onions and garlic for 1 minute. Add broccoli, stirring and cooking for about 2 minutes, or until coated. Reduce heat, add water, cover, and cook 3 minutes more. Remove cover and stir-fry a few more seconds. Add seasoning. Serve immediately.

In general, all vegetables should be cooked like this: as little as possible. Raw and steamed are good options. Sautéing holds the flavor in. When vegetables are put in water to boil for the usual method of cooking, it is estimated that in 4 minutes half the vitamins and half the minerals have moved into the water.

Prep. time: 10 minutes    Calcium  ★ ★ ★        B vitamins  ★ ★
Serves 4                  Magnesium  ★ ★        Vitamin C  ★ ★ ★
                         Vitamin A   ★ ★ ★

### Holiday Carrots

    5 cups sliced carrots
    3 Tb. butter
    1 medium onion, sliced thin
    12 stuffed green olives

Steam or quick-fry the carrots. Sauté onions in the butter until clear. Slice olives. Put carrots in serving dish. Add onions and butter and olives. Use parsley or fine herbs instead of salt.

Olives are extremely high in sodium. Do not use added salt in this dish and balance the vegetable with a baked potato or other potassium-containing food.

Prep. time: 45 minutes          Vitamin A  ★ ★ ★ ★
Serves 6

### Orange-Almond Carrots

    1 lb. carrots sliced in 1-inch pieces
    ½ cup orange juice
    2 Tb. honey
    1 Tb. butter
    ½ tsp. salt
    ¼ tsp. lemon rind, grated
    ⅓ cup blanched slivered almonds
    ½ tsp. vitamin C crystals
    2 Tb. fresh parsley

Steam carrots for 15 to 20 minutes, until tender. Combine orange juice, honey, butter, salt, and rind. Bring to a boil. Simmer, covered, for 5 minutes. Remove carrots from steamer, add to sauce, stir in almonds, and heat through. Stir in vitamin C and garnish with parsley. Serve immediately.

Prep. time: 30 minutes    **Protein** ★ ★      **Vitamin C** ★ ★ ★ ★
Serves 4 to 6            **Calcium** ★ ★      Other: phosphorus,
                           **Magnesium** ★ ★ ★        iron, and
                           **Vitamin A** ★ ★ ★ ★       potassium

### Parsley Dumplings

1 cup whole wheat pastry flour
2 tsp. baking powder
½ tsp. salt
3 Tb. dehydrated parsley flakes
½ cup milk
2 Tb. salad oil

Combine and mix all dry ingredients including parsley. Add milk and oil. Stir until moist. Drop by the tablespoonful into bubbling stew. Cover. Let the mixture return to boiling and reduce heat. Do not remove the cover until done. Simmer 12 to 15 minutes.

Prep. time: 10 minutes            **Protein** ★ ★
Serves 4                     **Vitamin A** ★ ★ ★ ★
                                 **B vitamins** ★ ★ ★

### Steamed Greens À La Greque

1 to 2 lbs. of fresh kale, collard, mustard, chard or other greens
Juice of ½ lemon (at least)
2 Tb. olive or other salad oil
Fine herb seasoning

Cook as described below for steamed spinach. Drain and cut through greens with a knife, making bite-size pieces.

Season with juice of at least ½ a lemon and 2 Tb. of olive or other salad oil. Sprinkle with fine herb seasoning. Toss lightly to coat all leaves. Serve immediately.

Kale, collards, chard, and mustard usually take about 15 to 20 minutes to steam. Save the coarse stems to use later in casseroles.

Prep. time: 30 minutes
Serves 4 to 6

Vitamin A  ★ ★ ★ ★
Vitamin C  ★ ★ ★
Calcium  ★ ★ ★

### Kale and Onion Sauté

1 large bunch kale, washed and
   shredded
2 large onions, chopped
2 cloves garlic, finely minced
2 Tb. oil
2–3 Tb. red wine vinegar (optional)
1 Tb. whole wheat flour
Salt and pepper to taste

Wash and shred kale. Cut off thick, tough stems. Chop fine. Place leaves and stems in large saucepan and steam for 20 minutes, covered. Sauté onions and garlic in oil. When kale is ready, add it and juice to the sauté mixture and toss well to combine. The vinegar makes it tangy but should be added along with the flour to the sautéed onion before putting in the kale. Season.

Prep. time: 30 minutes
Serves 3 or 4

Calcium  ★ ★ ★
B vitamins  ★ ★

Vitamin A  ★ ★ ★
Vitamin C  ★ ★ ★

### Steamed Spinach

1 to 2 lbs. fresh spinach

Cut off coarse stems and pick over the leaves carefully. Wash in water 5 times. Put leaves into a deep saucepan or a small kettle that will just hold them and cover the pan or kettle tightly. Add no water; the water that clings to the leaves is sufficient to cook them. Cook over medium heat and shake pan several times. As soon as the leaves have wilted down to the bottom of the pan and are bright green, they are done (4 to 5 minutes). Drain well and serve. Season as desired.

Prep. time: 30 minutes     **Vitamin A**   ★ ★ ★ ★
Serves 4                **Iron**   ★ ★ ★
                             **B vitamins**   ★ ★

### Spinach Surprise

  2 boxes frozen chopped spinach
  ½ cup raisins
  ½ cup slivered almonds or shelled
     sunflower seeds
2½ Tb. butter
  2 Tb. brewer's yeast
  ½ tsp. seasoning

Steam spinach; drain thoroughly. Just before serving, stir in raisins, almonds, butter, yeast, and seasoning. Reheat a minute: it should be served hot.

Prep. time:      **Protein**   ★ ★ ★     **B vitamins**   ★ ★ ★ ★
30 minutes     **Calcium**   ★ ★ ★     Other: phosphorus,
Serves 8       **Magnesium**   ★ ★ ★       iron, and
              **Vitamin A**   ★ ★ ★ ★       potassium

### Recipes with High Amounts of Vitamin C

It is virtually impossible to get our recommended dosage of vitamin C in foods alone. You would be eating twenty oranges a day, which would be impractical, messy, expensive, and boring. That is why the vitamin C crystals are used, and the brand used for these recipes delivers 4000 mg of vitamin C per teaspoon.

Heat destroys vitamin C, but the crystals should be dissolved in a small amount of lukewarm liquid, then returned to the dish; this avoids the possibility of biting down on an undissolved crystal, which is *very* tart. Always keep a C-containing food covered, and consume all of it at one meal if possible. Sodium ascorbate is not as sour and the powder dissolves readily.

Since cooking decreases the vitamin C content 50 to 80 percent, you'll want your foods to be covered and cooked a minimum of time in about 25 percent of the normal water required. Cook broccoli covered in a small amount of water, just enough to keep from sticking, and serve crisp. Add the butter or seasoning to the water and pour over broccoli just before serving—or, better still, eat raw. Do not steam vitamin C-containing foods you wish to be cooked: boiling is less destructive of the C. (Steam and oxygen destroys vitamin C.)

Although citrus fruits are traditionally the best source of C, some sprouts contain six times the vitamin C (per weight) of an orange!

Growing your own sprouts is very easy and inexpensive. When seeds sprout, the food value in them increases enormously. Vitamin C appears in abundance, and other nutrients double or triple. Starches turn to sugar that is readily acceptable in the body.

Sprouts can be used in breads, soups, and stews as well as in salads and sandwiches. Almost any seed or bean not chemically treated for planting can be used.

The most popular sprouts to pep up a dish are alfalfa, mung beans, wheat berries, peas, lentils, garbanzos—as are radish or mustard seeds.

*Method:* Soak 1 Tb. of seeds or ⅓ cup beans in 1 qt. lukewarm water overnight. Next day, rinse thoroughly in tepid water and drain. Place drained beans in a quart jar, cover it with a dampened piece of muslin, and secure the cloth with a rubber band. Store in a dark cupboard; under the sink is ideal.

Rinse the seeds two or three times a day, being sure all moisture is drained off. On day three, growing sprouts will rise to the top of the rinse water. Discard any ungerminated seeds.

Usually the sprouts are perfect for use by the third day except for alfalfa, which may take a day or two longer. Shake the sprouts into clear cold water and untangle them. Let them drain in a colander in the sun for an hour or two to increase their food value and to give them a little color. Store in the refrigerator until used.

Soybean sprouts need special attention because they mold or sour easily. Be sure to remove unsprouted beans as soon as you see them and rinse the seeds three or more times a day. They should always be cooked before using because they contain an enzyme that inhibits absorption of protein. Steam them for five minutes and then use in any dish of your choice.

And green peppers, parsley, broccoli, and cabbage— even spinach and cauliflower—contain more C than an orange! Strawberries and papaya are also good sources. Be sure to choose firm fruit; bruised fruit contains less C. And the most vitamin retention will be achieved by washing briefly, cutting, and eating immediately. Again, cover all fruit salads or other dishes containing C and don't allow them to linger as leftovers.

If a sweetener is required for a dish, use honey. It is the best sweetener nutritionally, but is still a sugar and should be used in minimum quantities. Buy the raw dark honeys, not the clarified and processed ones you see often on the supermarket shelves.

Sources of fair amounts of vitamin C: alfalfa, burdock, boneset, catnip, cayenne, chickweed, dandelion, garlic, hawthorn berry, horseradish, kelp, papaya, parsley, plantain, red raspberry leaf, rose hips, strawberry leaf, watercress.

### SALADS

The fruit dishes in this section can also be used as desserts. The other recipes make satisfying lunches.

### Chilled Ambrosia

> 4 cups fresh orange sections
> 1 cup unsweetened coconut shreds
> ⅓ cup orange-pineapple juice
> ½ tsp. vitamin C crystals
> 1 Tb. honey

Combine all ingredients. Chill.

Prep. time: 15 minutes          **Vitamin C**  ★ ★ ★ ★
Serves 6

### Salmon Fruit Salad

> 1 cup canned salmon, boned, rinsed,
>    and drained
> ¼ cup unhulled sesame seeds
> ⅓ cup mayonnaise
> 3 Tb. apple juice concentrate,
>    warmed
> ½ tsp. vitamin C crystals dissolved in
>    the apple juice
> 2 cups unpeeled diced apples
> ½ cup raisins
> ½ cup broken walnuts
> ½ cup diced celery
> ¼ cup apple-juice concentrate

Combine salmon, sesame seeds, mayonnaise, and juice concentrate with vitamin C. Stir in apples, raisins, nuts, and celery. Pour ¼ cup juice concentrate over all.

Prep. time: 15 minutes    **Protein** ★ ★ ★      **Vitamin C** ★ ★ ★ ★
Serves 6                  **Calcium** ★ ★ ★ ★    **Other:** potassium
                            **Magnesium** ★ ★ ★         and
                            **B vitamins** ★ ★ ★      phosphorus

When fish is boned, the calcium is lost. It is best to flake the fish and mash the bone into the mixture.

### Spinach-Orange Salad

    1 10-oz. bunch fresh spinach
    2 cups fresh orange sections
    3 Tb. chopped green onion tops
    1 cup plain yogurt
    2 Tb. orange-juice concentrate
    1½ Tb. honey, warmed
    2 tsp. vitamin C crystals dissolved in
       the honey

Wash spinach thoroughly and drain. Stem and tear into large bowl and toss with orange sections and onion tops. Combine yogurt, juice, and honey mixture. Pour over salad just before serving.

Prep. time: 10 minutes    **Protein** ★ ★      **Vitamin A** ★ ★ ★ ★
Serves 4 to 6            **Calcium** ★ ★      **Vitamin C** ★ ★ ★ ★

### Sticks and Stones Salad

    2 cups shredded carrots
    1 apple, peeled and shredded
    2 apples, unpeeled and diced
    ¼ cup mayonnaise
    ¼ cup apple-juice concentrate
    ½ tsp. vitamin C crystals, dissolved in
       juice concentrate
    ½ tsp. lemon juice
    Dash salt
    ¾ cup raisins

Combine all ingredients except raisins. Stir well, cover, and chill. Add raisins just before serving.

Prep. time: 10 minutes

Serves 4

Vitamin A  ★ ★ ★

Vitamin C  ★ ★ ★ ★

Other: potassium and iron

### Sprouter Space Salad

4 cups wheat sprouts
2 large navel oranges
1 pink grapefruit
1 15-oz. can chunk pineapple in its
   own juice
1 cup raisins

Place sprouts in large bowl. Peel and section oranges and grapefruit and add to sprouts. Drain pineapple and slice each chunk in half. Add pineapple and raisins to salad. Moisten with honey-anise dressing (page 267).

Prep. time: 15 minutes

Serves 6

Protein  ★ ★ ★

B vitamins  ★ ★ ★

Vitamin C  ★ ★ ★ ★

Other: potassium
and iron

### Sunshine Salad

4 medium carrots
2 large apples, unpeeled
2 bananas, sliced
1 cup unsweetened crushed pineapple, drained
1 cup plain yogurt
1 Tb. lemon juice
1 Tb. honey
½ tsp. vitamin C crystals dissolved in
   1 Tb. warm water
1 cup alfalfa sprouts

Shred carrots and apples. Add bananas and stir in pineapple. Combine yogurt, lemon juice, honey, and dissolved vitamin C and blend with a fork or whisk until smooth. Gently fold dressing into salad; place in bowl and top with sprouts.

Prep. time: 15 minutes  **Protein** ★ ★ ★     **B vitamins** ★ ★ ★
Serves 6                **Calcium** ★ ★       **Vitamin C** ★ ★ ★ ★
                        **Vitamin A** ★ ★ ★   **Other:** potassium


### Tuna Salad

    2 6½-oz. cans tuna
    1 15½-oz. can unsweetened crushed
        pineapple, drained
    1 cup diced celery
    ½ cup broken nuts
    2 apples, unpeeled and diced
    2 pears, unpeeled and diced
    Dash salt
    Celery-seed dressing (page 266)

Rinse tuna in strainer with cold water; drain. Combine next 6 ingredients with tuna and cover with celery-seed dressing to taste. Mix well and refrigerate, covered, to blend flavors.

Prep. time: 20 minutes  **Protein** ★ ★ ★     **B vitamins** ★ ★ ★
Serves 6 to 8           **Calcium** ★ ★ ★     **Vitamin C** ★ ★ ★
                        **Magnesium** ★ ★ ★

# Sweetness, 13 Love, and Special Desserts

Most of us love sweet things; some of us crave sweet things. A craving is revealed when the possessed person arises at 2 A.M. and eats a whole box of brown sugar. The good Lord gave us sweet-detecting taste buds hooked up to the pleasure center in our brain so we would love breast milk, which is very sweet, and fruit. We don't like unripe fruit (too sour) or rotten fruit. When it tastes sweet it has more vitamin C than at any other time; the forces of nature want us to eat the fruit at that particular time so we won't get scurvy.

We should try to satisfy our sweet taste with fruit, but it would be best to eat some protein or complex carbohydrate along with it since the quick sugar can produce the highs and lows we want to avoid. This is one reason why cheese and fruit are often served together.

The following sweet-tasting recipes are to be used for rare occasions. There are enough good nutrients to justify their inclusion in this book, but try to confine their use to parties and anniversaries. We must not teach our children that a sweet dessert follows every meal.

Vitamin C as a powder usually comes as 4000 mg per teaspoonful. Dissolve a teaspoonful in a tablespoon of warm water and add to most all of these recipes (this also controls some of the oxidation that fruits go through when exposed to the air).

One of the best first foods for the baby at about nine to eleven months could be a mashed banana sprinkled with brewer's yeast. It is prudent to have brewer's yeast powder, vitamin C powder, and dolomite (watch out for trace metals in compound; they can be contaminants) available in kitchen containers to be thrown into recipes—in appropriate amounts in appropriate dishes—for specific conditions. Yeast would be good for the tired, moody, depressed, or Jekyll-and-Hyde type who craves sugar. Vitamin C would be available as soon as the parents noted a cold, the flu, or a flareup of allergy symptoms. The calcium and magnesium could be added to dishes for the child who seems hyperactive, restless, or cannot relax and sleep.

Sweetness is love, but it can be nutritious love.

**Sugar Replacements**

Barley malt extract
Apple juice
Apple-juice concentrate (frozen, unsweetened)
Dried fruits cooked in a small amount of water, then
    ground with the liquid in which they were cooked
Grain coffees
Herbal teas
Chestnut flour
Nut butters
Fruit sugars (date, grape, etc.)
Honey—if you *must;* raw is better than others

Pan-roasting cereals will add sweetness and add the browned look usually associated with sugar. *To pan roast:* Place grains or flour in a heavy skillet and heat over low-medium heat, stirring constantly until the desired color is attained.

## Dessert or Snack Drinks

### Banana Milkshake

½ cup sesame milk
½ cup orange juice
1 frozen banana
1 Tb. wheat germ
2 or 3 ice cubes

Combine all ingredients in blender. Cover and process until smooth.

Prep. time: 3 minutes
Yield: 2 cups

Protein ★ ★ ★
Calcium ★ ★ ★
Other: potassium

### Almond Piña Colada Nog

12 almonds, ground
¾ cup crushed pineapple, unsweetened (canned)
1 heaping tsp. unsweetened coconut, shredded
3 or 4 crushed ice cubes
½ cup apple, orange, or pineapple juice

Grind almonds in blender and add remaining ingredients. Blend until ice dissolves

Prep. time: 10 minutes
Serves 2

Protein ★ ★
Calcium ★ ★
Vitamin C ★ ★ ★

### Mock Chocolate Shake

½ cup apple juice
½ banana
1 heaping tsp. carob powder
4 ice cubes
2 heaping tsp. shelled sunflower
  seeds
1 egg (optional)

Blend all ingredients until ice disappears and drink is foamy.

Prep. time: 5 minutes          Protein   ★ ★
Serves 1                       Calcium   ★ ★

### Apricot Pineapple Nog

1 cup cold pineapple juice, unsweetened
2 heaping Tb. apricot butter or
  chopped, dry apricots
1 egg (optional)
½ banana (optional)
3 ice cubes

Blend all ingredients until ice disappears and drink is foamy.

Prep. time: 5 minutes   Protein   ★ ★       Vitamin C   ★ ★
Serves 2                Vitamin A   ★ ★ ★    Other: potassium

### Rocky's Punch

1 cup crushed canned pineapple, unsweetened, undrained
½ cup apple juice
2 Tb. sunflower seeds, shelled
1 tsp. carob powder
1 Tb. brewer's yeast
3 ice cubes
2 eggs (optional)
2 tsp. blackstrap molasses

Put all ingredients in blender except molasses. Drizzle that in last, then blend until ice disappears and drink is foamy.

Prep. time: 5 minutes    **Protein** ★ ★ ★    **B vitamins** ★ ★
Serves 2    **Calcium** ★ ★ ★    **Vitamin C** ★ ★ ★

## CAKES, PIES, AND FROSTINGS

### Zucchini Bread

   3 eggs, beaten
   ¾ cup oil
   1¾ cups honey or sugar substitute
   2½ cups grated zucchini
   2 tsp. vanilla
   1 tsp. salt
   1 tsp. cinnamon
   1 tsp. soda
   ¼ tsp. baking powder
   4 cups whole wheat flour

Combine all ingredients in order given. Pour into 2 greased loaf pans. Bake in preheated 325° oven for 45 minutes, lower to 250°, and continue to bake for 15 minutes more.

Cut down the honey by ⅛ to ¼ cup the second time.

Prep. time: 30 minutes    **Protein** ★ ★    **B vitamins** ★ ★ ★
Yield: 2 loaves    **Vitamin A** ★ ★    **Other: potassium**

### No-Wheat Pie Crust

   2 cups flour—equal parts rice, soy,
     and potato
   ¾ tsp. salt
   ⅔ cup sunflower seed oil
   3 Tb. nut milk (or soy milk or permis-
     sible milk)

Combine flour and salt in a 9- or 10-inch pie pan. Add oil and liquid. Stir with a fork until the mixture is moist.

Remove ⅓ of the mixture for top crust. Press the remaining mixture over bottom and sides of pan. Fill bottom crust with fruit. Crumble the remaining ⅓ of the flour mixture over the surface of the filling. Bake in preheated 400° oven for 15 minutes. Lower the heat to 350° and bake until filling is cooked.

Prep. time: 30 minutes     **Protein** ★ ★ ★
Serves 6 to 8     **B vitamins** ★ ★ ★

### Carrot Cake

| | |
|---|---|
| 1½ cups safflower oil | ¾ tsp. salt |
| 1 cup honey | 1½ tsp. soda |
| 4 eggs | 1 tsp. allspice |
| 1 cup whole wheat flour | 2¼ cups shredded carrots |
| ¼ cup wheat germ | ½ cup chopped walnuts |
| ¼ cup soy flour, sifted | |

Mix oil, honey, and eggs until well blended. Add dry ingredients; blend thoroughly. Stir in carrots and nuts, then turn into well-greased and floured 6½-by-10-inch pan. Bake in preheated 350° oven 40 to 45 minutes. Cool for a few minutes, then invert on rack for at least 30 minutes. Frost with cream-cheese icing, if desired.

Prep. time: 1 hour    **Protein** ★ ★     **Vitamin A** ★ ★ ★
Serves 8    **Calcium** ★ ★     **B vitamins** ★ ★ ★
   **Magnesium** ★ ★

### Cream-Cheese Icing

10 oz. cream cheese at room tempera-
    ture
1 Tb. plain yogurt
1 tsp. vanilla
⅛ to ¼ cup honey

Whip cheese on high mixer speed until very fluffy. Add yogurt and vanilla. Beat until very smooth. Add honey in a steady stream while mixer is running, adding until frosting reaches desired consistency.

Prep. time: 5 minutes              Protein   ★ ★ ★
Yield: 1½ cups icing—enough for    Calcium   ★ ★ ★
    top and sides of 6½-by-
    10-inch cake


### Valentine's Day Sweetheart Cherry Pie

*Crust*

   2 cups stone-ground whole wheat
     flour
2½ tsp. salt-free baking powder
   3 Tb. safflower oil
   ⅔ cup water

Sift together flour and baking powder. Cut oil into flour mixture until it looks like large crumbs. Add water and stir to moisten flour. Knead dough for 1 minute on lightly floured board. Roll dough ¼ to ½ inch thick. Line pie pan with dough and fill with cherry filling.

*Cherry Filling*

1-lb. bag frozen unsweetened bing
   cherries
1 cup unsweetened apple juice
1 6-oz. can frozen pineapple concentrate, thawed
1 tsp. lemon juice

Mix together all ingredients. Bring to a boil. Lower heat and simmer until mixture is quite thick, about 30 minutes. Stir often. Cool and pour into crust. Bake in preheated 350° oven for an hour, or until crust is browned. Serve with blueberry sherbet. (page 262).

Prep. time: 50 minutes       Protein   ★ ★ ★
Serves 6 to 8                Vitamin A   ★ ★
                      B vitamins   ★ ★ ★

### No-Chocolate Syrup and Frosting

8 Tb. carob powder
3 cups water
¼ tsp. salt
2 Tb. soybean flour
½ cup currants, raisins, or chopped
   dates
1 Tb. arrowroot
1 Tb. Pero or decaffeinated coffee
1 tsp. vanilla extract

Mix carob in water to make a smooth paste. Add salt and bring to a boil. Reduce heat and simmer for 15 minutes. Add soybean flour gradually, beating with a whisk or eggbeater. Add fruit and continue simmering for 15 minutes, covered. Remove about ¼ cup of the carob mixture and stir the arrowroot into it. Add the Pero or coffee to make a smooth paste. Add this to the pan and stir until thick. Cool slightly and liquify in a blender. Good as a topping for puddings and cakes. Can be thickened by adding 2 to 4 Tb. tahini (sesame) or almond butter and used as a frosting.

Prep. time: 45 minutes          **Protein**  ★ ★
Yield: 2½ cups                   **Calcium**  ★ ★
                                 **Other: potassium and iron**

### Hot Peach Treat

1 cup millet
3 cups water
1 cup diced dried peaches
2 Tb. honey
1 Tb. butter or margarine
½ tsp. salt
1 cup plain yogurt

Just before retiring at night, bring millet, water, and peaches to a boil, then cover and refrigerate. In the morning, bring to a boil, covered, and cook gently on medium heat for 10 minutes or until water is absorbed. Stir in honey, butter, salt, and yogurt, mixing until creamy. Serve hot.

Prep. time: 10 minutes   Vitamin A  ★ ★ ★   Protein  ★ ★ ★
            overnight     B vitamins  ★ ★ ★  Calcium  ★ ★
Serves 4 to 6            Other: iron            Magnesium  ★ ★

## CANDIES

### Almond Coconut Apricots

¾ cup grated almonds
¼ cup honey
1 cup unsweetened shredded coconut
½ to 1 lb. dried apricot halves

Chop almonds in blender a few at a time until you have ¾ cup. Mix almonds, honey, and coconut. Form into 1-inch balls and place on apricot halves, flattening them slightly.

Prep. time: 30 minutes       Protein  ★ ★ ★
Yield: 2 dozen               Magnesium  ★ ★ ★
                             Vitamin A  ★ ★ ★ ★
                             Other: potassium and iron

### Apricot Candy

⅓ cup grated unsweetened coconut
¾ cup chopped nuts (almonds, pecans,
   or walnuts)
1 tsp. each lemon juice, grated lemon
   rind, and orange juice
¾ cup dried apricots, steamed 5 minutes in ½ cup water and drained
½ cup wheat germ

Use blender to blend, then shape into balls and roll in wheat germ.

Prep. time: 30 minutes   **Protein**  ★ ★        **B vitamins**  ★ ★
Yield: 2 dozen           **Vitamin A**  ★ ★ ★ ★   **Vitamin C**  ★ ★

### Carob Balls

½ cup carob powder
½ cup honey (optional) or barley malt
  extract
½ cup natural peanut butter
½ cup shelled sunflower seeds
½ cup unhulled sesame seeds
¼ cup wheat germ or shelled pumpkin seeds
¼ cup soy grits or soy flour
½ cup unsweetened coconut crumbs
  or ground nutmeats

Combine all ingredients except coconut or nutmeats. Form
into balls and roll in unsweetened coconut or nuts.

Prep. time: 20 minutes   **Protein**  ★ ★ ★     **B vitamins**  ★ ★ ★
Yield: 3 dozen           **Calcium**  ★ ★ ★     **Other:** phosphorus
                         **Magnesium**  ★ ★ ★

### Fruit Candy

¾ cup dried figs, chopped
½ cup ground nuts (walnuts, almonds,
  or pecans)
1 tsp. lemon juice
1 tsp. grated lemon peel or orange
  peel
¾ cup ground coconut, wheat germ, or
  unhulled sesame seeds

Combine first 4 ingredients. Make into balls and roll in the
coconut, wheat germ, or unhulled sesame seeds.

Prep. time: 30 minutes   **Protein**  ★ ★       **Vitamin C**  ★ ★
Yield: 2 dozen           **B vitamins**  ★ ★    **Other:** potassium

### Coconut Candy

    1 cup natural-style peanut butter
    1 cup seedless raisins
    ½ cup honey (or less)
    1 tsp. vanilla
    1½ cups unsweetened coconut, shredded

Combine first 4 ingredients. Spread the coconut on a flat pan or waxed paper. Drop spoonfuls of the peanut mixture onto the coconut and roll to coat them. Chill.

Prep. time: 30 minutes
Yield: 2 dozen

Protein ★★★★
Calcium ★★
B vitamins ★★★
Other: potassium and iron

### Filled Coconut Figs

    1 lb. or more dark figs
    ½ lb. almonds or filberts
    ½ cup honey
    1 tsp. lemon juice
    1 cup toasted or plain unsweetened
      shredded coconut

Stem figs. Slit and stuff each fig with one or two nuts. Put aside. Warm honey and lemon juice together. Stir in figs until well coated. Then roll in coconut to coat well.

Prep. time: 20 minutes
Yield: 2 to 3 dozen

Protein ★★★
Magnesium ★★★
B vitamins ★★★
Other: potassium, phosphorus,
      and iron

### Peanut Butter Balls

½ cup natural-style peanut butter
1 cup nonfat milk powder
¼ cup fruit preserves (strawberry,
    cherry, pineapple)
½ cup unsweetened coconut, wheat
    germ, or ground unsalted nuts if de-
    sired

Mix together first 3 ingredients. Form into 1-inch balls. Roll in coconut, wheat germ, or ground unsalted nuts.

Prep. time: 20 minutes       **Protein**  ★ ★ ★ ★
Yield: 2 dozen               **Calcium**  ★ ★ ★
                            **B vitamins**  ★ ★ ★

## COOKIES

### Applets

2 Tb. plain gelatin
½ cup cold apple juice
2 cups unsweetened applesauce
1½ cups chopped salt-free nuts

Dissolve gelatin in apple juice. Mix with other ingredients and put in an oiled pan to firm (about 2 hours). Cut into 1-inch squares and dust with fructose or finely chopped nuts.

Prep. time: 10 minutes/2 hrs    **Protein**  ★ ★ ★
Yield: 3 dozen                 **Magnesium**  ★ ★ ★

### Date-Nut Bars

3 eggs, slightly beaten          1 cup whole wheat flour
2 cups dates, pitted             ½ cup honey
1 cup walnuts or almonds         ½ cup bran (or ¼ cup bran
1 tsp. baking powder                 and ¼ cup wheat germ)

Combine eggs with all other ingredients. Line a 9-by-13-inch pan with waxed paper. Spread batter in pan. (It looks as if it will never cover the dates and nuts, but it tends to spread and rise as it bakes.) Bake 45 minutes in preheated 250° oven. Remove from oven and cool 10 minutes. Invert pan and peel off waxed paper. Cool 20 minutes, then cut into rectangular bars. Store in airtight container.

Prep. time: 30 minutes　　　Protein　★ ★ ★
Yield: 2 dozen　　　　　　　Magnesium　★ ★ ★
　　　　　　　　　　　　　　B vitamins　★ ★ ★
　　　　　　　　　　　　　　Other: potassium and phos-
　　　　　　　　　　　　　　　　　phorus

### Banana and Raisin Cookies

　3 bananas, mashed
　½ cup chopped nuts (pecans, walnuts,
　　almonds)
　⅓ cup vegetable oil
　1 cup chopped raisins
　½ tsp. salt
　1 tsp. vanilla
　2 cups oatmeal

Mix all ingredients and let stand until moisture is absorbed. Drop by small spoonfuls on ungreased cookie sheet. Bake in preheated 350° oven for 20 to 25 minutes.

Prep. time: 1 hour　　　　　Protein　★ ★
Yield: 3 dozen　　　　　　　B vitamins　★ ★ ★
　　　　　　　　　　　　　　Other: potassium and iron

### Daties

　½ cup honey　　　　　　　　¼ tsp. salt
　2 eggs　　　　　　　　　　　1 cup chopped dates
　½ cup whole wheat flour　　1 cup chopped walnuts
　1 Tb. dolomite powder　　　½ cup unsweetened coconut
　½ tsp. baking powder

Beat honey and eggs until smooth; add next 6 ingredients and mix well. Spoon batter into greased square 9-by-9-inch pan and bake for 20 minutes in preheated 350° oven. Remove from oven and stir immediately. Cool 5 to 10 minutes. With buttered hands, roll cooked mixture into balls, then roll in coconut. Cool completely, then store in a tightly covered container in a cool place.

Prep. time: 1 hour     Protein  ★ ★ ★        B vitamins  ★ ★ ★
Yield: 3 dozen         Calcium  ★ ★ ★        Other: potassium
                       Magnesium  ★ ★ ★            and iron

## SNACKS

### Cannonballs

    1 box golden raisins
    1 cup roasted peanuts
    1 6-oz. bag dried apricots
    ½ cup unhulled sesame seeds

Chop raisins, peanuts, apricots, and sesame seeds, alternating in that order, using fine blade of food chopper. Mix well with hands, roll into balls, and store, covered, in refrigerator.

Prep. time: 20 minutes   Protein  ★ ★ ★      B vitamins  ★ ★ ★
Yield: 3 dozen           Calcium  ★ ★ ★      Other: potassium
                        Magnesium  ★ ★ ★
                        Vitamin A  ★ ★ ★ ★

### Homemade Crackerjacks

    ¼ cup honey
    ¼ cup butter or margarine
    1½ quarts popped popcorn
    ¾ cup peanuts (shelled)

Melt honey and butter or margarine in a small saucepan. Place popped corn and peanuts in a large bowl and mix together. Add the honey mixture and stir to completely coat the popcorn and peanuts. Spread the mixture in a single layer on a cookie sheet (you will have to make several batches). Bake 10 to 15 minutes in preheated 350° oven or until crisp. Cool in large bowl and store in tightly covered container.

Prep. time: 1 hour
Yield: 2 quarts

Protein  ★★
Vitamin A  ★★★
B vitamins  ★★★


### Banana Crunchies

¾ cup orange juice
3 bananas
½ cup chopped salt-free nuts or wheat
    germ

Peel and cut bananas into 1-inch slices. Using a fork, dip in juice, then roll in nuts or wheat germ. May be frozen.

Prep. time: 15 minutes    Protein  ★★      B vitamins  ★★
Yield: 20 pieces          Vitamin C  ★★    Other: potassium


### Date and Apple Tidbits

¾ cup water
¾ cup frozen unsweetened apple-juice
    concentrate
7 whole cloves
¼ tsp. ginger
½ tsp. cinnamon
6 apples, peeled and sliced or
    chopped
1 cup dates, pitted and chopped

Combine juice concentrate and spices in a large saucepan and bring to a boil. While boiling, add the apples and cook

until soft. Add dates and cook 10 minutes more. Add more
water if needed. Can be used on French toast, waffles,
pancakes, muffins, and the like.

Prep. time: 40 minutes          **B vitamins**  ★ ★
Serves 6                        **Other: potassium**


### Trail Mix

6 pieces dried honey-coated papaya,
   chopped
½ lb. dried banana chips
¼ cup dried chopped pineapple
¼ cup dried chopped apricots
½ lb. dry roasted almonds
¼ lb. dry roasted cashews
1 cup dried unsweetened coconut
   shavings
1 cup chopped dates
1 cup carob chips
1 cup shelled sunflower seeds

Mix all ingredients in a bowl. Store in tightly covered
container in a cool place.

Prep. time: 15 minutes          **Protein**  ★ ★ ★
Yield: 6½ cups                  **Magnesium**  ★ ★ ★
                                **Vitamin A**  ★ ★ ★

Some find this too sweet. Eliminate items one and two and
the carob. Use raisins, filberts, brazil nuts, and pumpkin
seeds.


### Toasted Pumpkin Seeds

Wash dried pumpkin seeds and soak overnight in salt
water. Pat dry. Spread thinly on cookie sheet and toast in
250° oven for 2 to 3 hours, stirring occasionally.

**Protein**  ★ ★ ★
**Other: phosphorus**

### Pumpkin-Seed Variation

1 cup seeds (after soaking)
2 Tb. Worcestershire sauce
2 Tb. melted butter or margarine
2 Tb. grated Parmesan cheese

Toss all ingredients together and roast in 250° oven for 2 hours.

Prep. time: 10 minutes          **Protein** ★★★
Yield: 1 cup                    **Calcium** ★★
                                **Other:** phosphorus

### Tutti Frutti

½ lb. prunes
½ lb. dried figs
 1 lb. pitted dates
 1 lb. seeded raisins
¼ lb. dried apricots
 2 cups walnut meats
½ cup shelled sunflower seeds
½ cup shelled, unsalted pumpkin
    seeds
Unsweetened coconut shreds (op-
    tional)

Pit prunes and stem figs. Put all ingredients except coconut in blender or food processor. Blend or grind until thoroughly mixed. Store tightly covered in refrigerator. May be rolled into balls and coated with coconut or thinned slightly with fruit juice and used as a sauce. Can be mixed with peanut butter for sandwich filling.

Prep. time: 30 minutes   **Protein** ★★★      **B vitamins** ★★★
Yield: 5¼ pounds         **Calcium** ★★       **Other:** potassium,
                        **Magnesium** ★★★          phosphorus,
                        **Vitamin A** ★★★          and iron

### PUDDINGS, SHERBETS, AND POPS

#### Carrot Pudding

1 cup whole wheat flour
¼ tsp. salt
1 tsp. soda
½ tsp. cinnamon
½ tsp. allspice
¼ tsp. cloves
1 cup grated peeled raw potato
1 cup grated raw carrots
½ cup melted shortening
¾ cup honey
1 cup raisins
½ cup chopped nuts

Sift dry ingredients together. Combine with carrots and potatoes. Add shortening, honey, raisins, and nuts. Mix well and put in greased pan. Steam 3½ hours. Serve with lemon juice.

Prep. time: 30 minutes     Protein   ★ ★
Serves 6     Vitamin A   ★ ★
    B vitamins   ★ ★
    Other:   potassium and iron

#### Sampan Pudding

1½ cups tofu, drained and crumbled
½ cup crunchy peanut butter
1½ bananas
Juice of ½ lemon or 2 Tb.
3-4 ice cubes
1½ Tb. honey
1 Tb. carob powder (optional)
1 Tb. unsweetened shredded coconut as garnish (optional)

Combine all ingredients except optional coconut in a blender and purée until smooth or until ice disappears.

Pour into sherbet glasses or dessert dishes and chill. Add coconut before serving.

*Variation:* Freeze until mixture begins to crystallize. Stir and serve.

Prep. time: 10 minutes      **Protein** ★ ★ ★
Serves 2 to 4


### Banana Sherbet

> 3 ripe bananas
> 1 lb. can crushed pineapple
> 1 6-oz. can frozen orange-juice con-
>    centrate
> ½ cup powdered milk

Whip all ingredients in blender until smooth. Pour into freezer trays and freeze until mushy. Whip again and freeze until firm.

Prep. time: 10 minutes      **Protein** ★ ★
           plus freezing time      **Calcium** ★ ★ ★
Serves 6                     **Vitamin C** ★ ★ ★
                            **Other: potassium**


### Blueberry Sherbet

> 1 package unflavored gelatin
> ⅔ cup unsweetened pineapple juice,
>    divided
> 1 6-oz. can frozen pineapple concen-
>    trate
> ¾ lb. fresh or unsweetened frozen
>    blueberries (picked over)
> 3 Tb. fresh lemon juice

Soften gelatin in ⅓ cup warm pineapple juice. Chill. Put gelatin mixture and all other ingredients into blender. Blend 5 minutes. Strain. Pour into ice-cube trays, using dividers. Freeze. Just before serving, put sherbet cubes and ⅓ cup chilled pineapple juice into blender. Blend until smooth. Serve on top of cherry pie.

Prep. time: 15 minutes          **Vitamin C**  ★ ★ ★
Serves 6 to 8


### Finger Jello

　　1 12-oz. can frozen juice concentrate
　　　(orange, apple, pear, grape)
　　3 envelopes unflavored gelatin
　　1½ cups (1 juice can) water

Soften gelatin in juice. Boil water and add juice mixture gradually, stirring until gelatin is dissolved. Remove from heat and pour into lightly greased 9-by-13-inch pan. Chill. Cut into squares when firm. Refrigerate.

Prep. time: 30 minutes          **Protein**  ★ ★ ★
Yield: 100 little squares        **Vitamin C**  ★ ★ ★


### Frozen Banana Pops

　　6 firm bananas
　　⅛ cup honey
　　⅓ cup lukewarm water
　　½ tsp. vitamin C crystals dissolved in
　　　water
　　½ cup granola crumbs or cinnamon
　　　toasties
　　6 wooden sticks or plastic skewers

Peel bananas, stick a skewer in the end of each one, and place in freezer for 30 minutes. Combine the honey and vitamin C mixture. Roll bananas in it, just to moisten, then roll in crumbs. Freeze until firm; store in plastic bag.

Prep. time: 10 minutes    **Protein**  ★ ★        **Vitamin C**  ★ ★ ★
　　　　　　plus freezing  **B vitamins**  ★ ★ ★  **Other: potassium**
Yield: 6 pops

### Yogurt Popsicles

2 cups plain yogurt
1 6-oz. can frozen orange-juice con-
     centrate
2 tsp. vanilla

Stir together. Freeze in small cups with sticks in middle.

Prep. time: 10 minutes plus                **Protein**   ★ ★
          freezing                         **Calcium**   ★ ★ ★
Yield: 15 popsicles                        **Vitamin C**   ★ ★ ★

# Nutritious 14
## Spreads, Dressings, and Dips

Spreads, seasonings, and dressings should be as nutritious as possible. Regular, store-bought catsup has more sugar than a soft drink; don't fool around with it.

### Basic Soup and Sauce Mix (for enrichment)

1½ cups powdered milk
1 cup soy flour
½ cup kelp powder
1 cup brewer's yeast

Combine all ingredients and keep refrigerated to use in soups and sauces. Add 3 Tb. of mixture to 1 cup of milk or other liquid when cooking.

Prep. time: 5 minutes
Yield: 4 cups

Calcium ★ ★
Protein ★ ★ ★
B vitamins ★ ★ ★
Many trace minerals

### Natural Catsup

1 12-oz. can tomato paste
½ cup cider vinegar
½ cup water
½ tsp. salt
1 tsp. oregano

⅛ tsp. cumin
⅛ tsp. nutmeg
⅛ tsp. pepper
½ tsp. mustard
⅛ tsp. garlic powder

Mix all ingredients thoroughly. Keep refrigerated.

Prep. time: 15 minutes
Yield: 1⅓ cups

**Vitamin A** ★ ★ ★
**Other: potassium and iron**

### Celery-Seed Dressing

1 egg
⅓ cup cider vinegar, lukewarm
½ tsp. vitamin C crystals dissolved in
   the vinegar
⅓ cup honey
2 Tb. celery seed
1 Tb. prepared mustard
1½ tsp. salt
1 tsp. paprika
1 cup safflower oil

Process first 8 ingredients in blender at high speed until blended. At low speed drizzle in oil until emulsified.

Prep. time: 5 minutes
Yield: 1½ cups

**Calcium** ★ ★ ★
**Vitamin C** ★ ★ ★ ★

### French Dressing

1½ cups safflower oil
¾ cup apple cider vinegar
¼ cup honey
2 Tb. brewer's yeast
1 Tb. minced onion
1½ tsp. salt
1 tsp. paprika
½ tsp. dry mustard
¼ tsp. black pepper

Process all ingredients in blender at high speed for 1 minute. Chill.

Prep. time: 5 minutes          B vitamins   ★ ★ ★
Yield: 2½ cups


### Honey-Anise Dressing

 4 oz. cream cheese, softened
½ cup plain yogurt
 1 Tb. honey, warmed
½ tsp. vitamin C crystals dissolved in
    honey
 1 Tb. lemon juice
½ tsp. anise seed

Combine all ingredients and whisk or beat until smooth. Cover and refrigerate to blend flavors. Serve with fruit salad.

Prep. time: 5 minutes          Protein   ★ ★ ★
Yield: 1¼ cups                  Calcium   ★ ★ ★
                               Vitamin C   ★ ★ ★ ★

There are no vitamins or minerals in this recipe worth recording, but it *is* a better, more healthful dressing than any of the commercial ones available at the store.


### Sour Cream Dressing

2 Tb. sour cream         1 tsp. dry mustard
2 cups safflower oil     ½ tsp. black pepper
⅓ cup white vinegar      1 tsp. fresh lemon juice
1 tsp. onion powder      ⅛ tsp. garlic powder

Mix together in a jar with a tight-fitting lid. Refrigerate. Could last a week or so.

Prep. time: 10 minutes
Yield: 2 cups

### Mayonnaise

2 eggs
2 Tb. vinegar, warmed
½ tsp. vitamin C crystals, dissolved in
    the vinegar
1 Tb. honey
½ tsp. salt
½ tsp. Dijon mustard
2 cups safflower oil
2 Tb. lemon juice

Place first 6 ingredients in blender and blend thoroughly. With the motor running, add half the oil in a thin steady stream. Add lemon juice. Drizzle in the remaining oil until emulsified. Store, covered, in refrigerator.

Prep. time: 5 minutes
Yield: 3 cups

**Protein**  ★ ★
**Vitamin A**  ★ ★
**Vitamin C**  ★ ★ ★ ★

### Wheatless Cream Sauce

¼ cup arrowroot, corn, or potato
    starch
1 Tb. dolomite, calcium lactate, or
    bone meal (optional)
¾ cup cold milk or nondairy milk
3½ cups scalded milk or nondairy
    milk
1 tsp. salt
½ tsp. white pepper
1 small onion, finely chopped

Dissolve starch and dolomite (optional) in cold milk, mixing well. Add hot milk and blend well. Add salt, pepper, and onion. Cook and stir over low heat for 15 minutes. Strain and use over vegetables, fish, chicken, or meat.

Prep. time: 20 minutes
Yield: 1 quart

**Protein**  ★ ★
**Calcium**  ★ ★

Freeze remainder for later use.

### Vegetarian Chopped Liver

1 Tb. oil
1 medium onion, sliced
1 lb. cooked green beans
½ cup chopped walnuts
2 hard-cooked eggs
Salt and pepper to taste
1 tsp. (or more) natural-style peanut
    butter

Sauté onion in heated oil until lightly browned. Using a meat grinder or food processer, grind the onion, beans, nuts, and eggs. Add peanut butter and chill. Serve on a bed of lettuce with whole wheat crackers or pita bread.

Prep. time: 30 minutes       **Protein**  ★ ★ ★
Serves 6                  **Magnesium**  ★ ★ ★
                           **B vitamins**  ★ ★ ★

### Peanut Butter–Tofu Spread

1 cup tofu, drained and crumbled
⅓ cup peanut butter
¾ banana
Juice of ½ lemon
1 Tb. honey
¼ to ½ cup hulled sunflower seeds,
    currants, raisins, or chopped nuts
    (optional)

Combine the first 5 ingredients in a blender or in a large bowl and beat or blend until smooth. Add the optional seeds, nuts, or currants. Serve as a spread on wholesome bread or crackers. Makes a delicious sandwich with the addition of sliced bananas, avocados, or apples. Good as a stuffing for celery or bok choy logs.

Prep. time: 10 minutes       **Protein**  ★ ★ ★
Serves 4                  **Calcium**  ★ ★

### Pineapple Dip

1 lb. dry-curd cottage cheese
1 8-oz. can unsweetened crushed
   pineapple

In a blender or by hand, mash the cheese until smooth. Add pineapple with its juice. Mix well.

Prep. time: 15 minutes
Yield: 3 cups

Protein ★★
Calcium ★★
Vitamin C ★★

### Tomato Dip

1 lb. dry-curd cottage cheese
1 cup salt-free tomato juice
1 tsp. onion powder
½ tsp. black pepper
4 drops Tabasco sauce

In a blender or by hand, mash the cheese until smooth. Add other ingredients. Mix well.

Prep. time: 15 minutes
Yield: 3 cups

Protein ★★
Calcium ★★
Vitamin A ★★★

### Tofu Dressing or Dip (Yaponeziki Skordalia)

7 oz. tofu, well drained and crumbled
Juice of 1 lemon
3 cloves garlic, minced
¼ to ½ tsp. salt or to taste
¼ to ½ tsp. dry mustard or to taste

Combine ingredients in blender and blend until smooth. Serve as a dip with fresh vegetables or crackers, as a dressing for salads, or as a sauce for cooked vegetables or fish. Delicious on baked potatoes. Use as mayonnaise on sandwiches.

Prep. time: 10 minutes
Yield: 1 cup

Protein ★★★

### Special Spread for Bread*

1 lb. margarine or butter
2 Tb. nonfat dry milk
1 cup safflower oil or sunflower oil
* May also be used in cooking.

Soften butter or margarine to room temperature and then add dry milk slowly while beating at medium speed. Next add the oil slowly. Keep refrigerated.

Prep. time: 5 minutes                    **Vitamin A**   ★ ★ ★ ★
Yield: 1½ lbs.

# Postscript: Recipe for Healthy Folk

1. Eat small amounts four to six times a day.

2. Eat raw fruit, vegetables, seeds, and nuts several times a day with and between meals. Eat enough so your bowel movements are on the edge of sloppiness.

3. Be as much of a vegetarian as you can.

4. Never have sugar, white flour, or boxed cereals in your house.

5. Dairy fat and animal fats are considered dangerous. Use low-fat, low-salt cheese. If you must eat beef, eat only two to three ounces every two weeks. (Eggs are now thought not to be so bad.)

6. You may have one dish of natural ice cream when the temperature rises above one hundred degrees.

7. Plan to live one hundred twenty years. Too many of us are locked into the idea that age seventy is it. Many animals live to be ten times their age at puberty. Why not us?

8. Walk or exercise daily, believe in a higher Being, say something nice about yourself and someone else daily.

272

# Bibliography

Allergy

Coca, Arthur. *The Pulse Test*. New York: Ace Publ. Co., A method of testing for food allergies.
Crook, William G. *Are You Allergic?* Jackson, Tenn.: Professional Books, 1978.
Crook, William G. *Tracking Down Hidden Food Allergy*. Jackson, Tenn.: Professional Books, 1978.
Frazier, Claude A. *Coping with Food Allergy*. New York: Quadrangle, 1974.
Rapp, Doris J. *Allergies and Your Child*. New York: Holt, Rinehart and Winston, 1972.


Diet and Behavior

Abrahamson, E. M. and A. W. Pezet. *Body, Mind, and Sugar*. New York: Avon, 1951.
Breneman, J. C. *Help Your Bed-Wetting Child*. Gales, Mich.: 1978.
Cheraskin, E., W. M. Ringsdorf, and A. Bresher. *Psychodietetics*. New York: Bantam Books, 1974.
Cott, Alan. *The Orthomolecular Approach to Learning Disabilities*. San Rafael, Calif.: Academic Therapy Publications, 1977.
Crook, William G. *Can Your Child Read? Is He Hyperactive?* Jackson, Tenn.: Professional Books, 1975.
Deutsch, R. M. *Realities of Nutrition*. Palo Alto, Calif.: Bull Publishing Co., 1976. A popularized approach exposing facts and fallacies and discusses the basis of present nutrition knowledge.
Dufty, William. *Sugar Blues*. New York: Chilton, 1975.
Goldbeck, Nikki and David. *The Supermarket Handbook: Access to Whole Foods*. New York: Harper & Row, 1973.
Feingold, B. F. *Why Your Child Is Hyperactive*. New York: Random House, 1974.

Hall, Ross Hume. *Food for Thought*. New York: Vintage Books, 1976.

Hunter, Beatrice T. *Consumer Beware! Your Food and What's Been Done to It*. New York: Simon & Schuster, 1971.

Hunter, Beatrice Trum. *Fact Book on Food Additives and Your Health*. New Canaan, Conn.: Keats Publishing, Inc., 1972.

Hyde, Margaret O. and Elizabeth Forsyth. *What Have You Been Eating? Do You Really Know?* New York: McGraw-Hill, 1975.

Jacobson, Michael F. *Eater's Digest: The Consumer's Factbook of Food Additives*. Garden City, N.Y.: Anchor Books, 1972.

La Leche League. *The Womanly Art of Breastfeeding*. Interstate Printers, 1958.

Lappe, Frances Moore. *Diet for a Small Planet*. New York: Ballantine Books, 1971.

Mackarness, Richard. *Eating Dangerously: The Hazards of Hidden Allergies*. New York: Harcourt Brace Jovanovich, 1976.

Null, Gary and Steven. *How to Get Rid of the Poisons in Your Body*. New York: Arco Publishing, 1977.

Oski, Frank A. *Don't Drink Your Milk*. Wyden Press, 1978.

Ott, John N. *Health and Light*. New York: Pocket Books, 1976.

Pryor, Karen. *Nursing Your Baby*. New York: Harper & Row, 1963.

Robertson, L., C. Flinders, and B. Godfrey. *Laurel's Kitchen: A Handbook for Vegetarian Cookery and Nutrition*. Petaluma, Calif.: Nilgiri Press, 1976.

Roth, June. *Cooking for Your Hyperactive Child*. Chicago: Contemporary Books, Inc., 1977.

Smith, Lendon H. *Improving Your Child's Behavior Chemistry*. Englewood Cliffs, N.J.: Prentice-Hall, 1976.

Speer, Fredrick. *Allergy of the Nervous System*. Springfield, Ill.: Charles C Thomas, 1970.

Stevens, George E., Laura J. Stevens, and Rosemary B. Stoner. *How to Feed Your Hyperactive Child*. Garden City, N.Y.: Doubleday, 1977.

Tannenbaum, Beulah and Myra Stillman. *Understanding Food*. New York: McGraw-Hill, 1962.

Wunderlich, Ray C. *Improving Your Diet*. St. Petersburg, Fla.: Johnny Reads, Inc., 1976.

## Cookbooks

Condas, Anastasia C. *More Junk Food Alternatives*. Castro Valley, Calif.: BEANS (Better Educational and Nutritional Standards) and CCRA (The Contra Costa Reading Association), 1979. Nutritional snacks and beverages without white flour and sugar.

Davis, Adelle. *Let's Cook It Right*. New York: Signet, 1947.

Dworkin, Stan and Floss. *The Good Goodies: Recipes for Natural Snacks 'n' Sweets*. Emmaus, Pa.: Rodale Press, 1974.

Emerling, Carol G. and Jonckers, Eugene O. *The Allergy Cookbook*. New York: Barnes & Noble, 1969.

Farmilant, Eunice. *The Natural Foods Sweet-Tooth Cookbook*. Garden City, N.Y.: Doubleday, 1973.

Kees, Beverly. *Cook with Honey*. Brattleboro, Vt.: The Stephen Greene Press, 1973.

Kinderlehrer, Jane. *Confessions of a Sneaky Organic Cook*. Emmaus, Pa.: Rodale Press, 1971.

Little, Billie. *Recipes for Allergies*. New York: Grosset & Dunlap, 1971.

Opton, Gene and Nancie Hughes. *Honey Feast*. San Francisco, Calif.: Apple Pie Press, 1974.

Shattuck, Ruth R. *Creative Cooking without Wheat, Milk and Eggs*. Cranbury, N.J.: A. S. Barnes, 1974.

Vaughan, Beatrice. *Real Old-Time Yankee Maple Cooking*. Brattleboro, Vt.: The Stephen Greene Press, 1969.

Other Sources of Information

Allergy Awareness Newsletter
Marilyn Sondy, Editor
1609 Mills Avenue
North Muskegon, Mich. 49445

An interesting, informal newsletter written by a dedicated mother of an allergic family.

Allergy Information Association
Room 7, 25 Poynter Drive
Weston, Ontario, Canada M9R 1K8

This is a superb volunteer organization dedicated to helping allergy sufferers. They are also concerned with the relationship of diet to behavior. They publish an interesting newsletter and offer helpful recipes.

Association for Children with Learning Disabilities (ACLD)
5225 Grace Street
Pittsburgh, Pa. 15236

The purpose of this national organization is to improve the educational opportunities of children with learning disabilities.

Center for Science in the Public Interest (CSPI)
1755 S Street, N.W.
Washington, D.C. 20009

The goal of this organization is to improve the quality of American diets through research and public education. They have several posters available. One poster, "Chemical Cuisine," is a handy guide to food additives. Another, "Nutrition Scoreboard," grades many foods according to their nutritional value. They also publish *Nutrition Action Magazine*.

The Feingold Association
56 Winston Drive
Smithtown, N.Y. 11787

This volunteer group of parents tries to help other parents of hyperactive and learning disabled children through a newsletter and local groups.

New York Institute for Child Development
205 Lexington Ave.
New York, N.Y. 10016

This organization publishes an informative newsletter, "Reading Children," about diet, behavior, and learning disabilities. They have some fascinating cassette tapes available.

Prevention Magazine
Emmaus, Pa. 18049

A monthly magazine devoted to better health through proper diet.

## FREE GOVERNMENT BOOKLETS

The booklets listed below are yours for the asking from Consumer Information Center, Pueblo, Colorado 81009. Be sure to include the *number* of the item you are requesting.

### Learning Activities for Children

*Good Food News for Kids*, #528H (1978). Games and puzzles to teach children about food; a package of four illustrated booklets that introduces the basic food groups to your children: *Meet Fred, the Horse Who Likes Bread* explains how bread gets from the farmer's field to your toaster. Fred tells what's so great about bread. There's also *Gussie Goose*, who introduces the fruit and vegetable group; *Mary Mutton*, who teaches your children about meat; and *Molly Moo*, who recommends dairy products.

*The Thing the Professor Forgot*, #531H (1978). A coloring book that teaches the importance of good nutrition and a well-balanced diet through pictures and rhyme and Professor Oonose Q. Eckwoose. He climbs into the pantry, finds his book behind a jam jar, and cautions "If you're going to be smart, be clever or shrewd, be sure to know there are four groups of food." Each food group has pictures to be colored.

### Nutrition for Everyone

*The Confusing World of Health Foods*, #534H (1979). Discusses the claims for health, organic, and natural foods. It compares cost and nutritional value of health versus conventional foods.

*Food*, #544H (1979). A hassle-free guide to a better diet that includes the truth about snacking, a nutritional case for breakfast, and quick and easy recipes with calorie counts and illustrations.

*Food Additives*, #545H (1979). Tells why chemicals are added to foods, how additive use is regulated, and steps to take to exert control over what goes into your food. Gives definitions of the major categories of additives and has an index of more than 130 additives.

*Grandma Called It Roughage*, #546H (1979). Contains claims and facts about high-fiber diets, effects on health, and food sources of fiber.

*A Primer on Dietary Minerals*, #548H (1978). Describes the necessary minerals and gives the best food sources for them.

*Proteins, Carbohydrates, Fats and Fibers*, #549 (1979). Tells what they are, what they do, and which are the best food sources.

*Some Facts and Myths About Vitamins*, #550H (1979). Explains what vitamins are, how they work, and gives the best food sources. Also examines some popular and controversial claims about vitamins.

### Preparation and Storage of Food for Better Nutrition

*Beginner's Guide to Home Canning and Freezing*, #642H (1977). Contains tips for selecting, preparing, and processing fruits and vegetables and a glossary.

*Can Your Kitchen Pass the Food Storage Test?*, #551H (1978). Contains a checklist of food-storage hazards and tells how to correct them.

*Food Safety for the Family*, #552H (1977). Has tips on preventing food poisoning and includes storage times and cooking temperatures for meat and poultry.

*Home Food Preservation*, #648H (1977). A how-to guide for home canning, freezing, and drying fruits and vegetables that includes making jellies, jams, and preserves (but you can skip those parts). Describes how to pickle, make wine, and store fresh fruits and vegetables. Includes a glossary.

*No-Nitrite Meats: Handle Carefully*, #554H (1979). Tells how to prepare and store uncured bologna, bacon, and frankfurters to protect against food poisoning.

*Safe Brown Bag Lunches*, #555H (1977). Suggests types of food best suited for packed lunches and discusses the precautions necessary to assure wholesomeness.

### Purchasing Food for Better Nutrition

*Consumer's Guide to Food Labels*, #558H (1978). Discusses ingredient and nutrient listings, open dating, metric units, and symbols used on food labels.

*How to Use USDA Grades in Buying Foods*, #560H (1979). Explains U.S. Department of Agriculture symbols to look for when buying meat, poultry, produce, butter, eggs, and so forth.

*Read the Label, Set a Better Table*, #561 (1976). Tells how to use nutrition labels to save money and serve balanced meals. It includes a chart of U.S. Recommended Daily Allowances and lists major food sources for each nutrient.

*Your Money's Worth in Foods*, #562 (1977). Contains guides for budgeting, menu planning, and shopping for best values.

### Gardening for Better Nutrition

*Fruits and Nuts*, #563 (1977). An illustrated guide for selecting, planting, and maintaining fruit trees, nut trees, and berry plants.

*Growing Vegetables in Containers*, #564H (1977). Types of containers, soil, planting techniques, and care of vegetable minigardens.

*Growing Your Own Vegetables*, #565H (1977). Everything you need to know about planning, planting, and caring for more than forty different kinds of vegetables.

*Herbs*, #566H (1977). Describes growing, drying, and freezing seventeen varieties of herbs; also contains basic recipes.

*Organic Gardening—Think Mulch*, #568 (1977). Growing crops without chemical fertilizers or pesticides, using organic mulches and fertilizers, and starting a compost heap.

*Year-Round Gardening With a Greenhouse*, #569H (1978). Where to get building plans for a greenhouse; how to heat, ventilate, and shade it; how to plant and cultivate flowers and tomatoes; and what the best plant varieties are for greenhouses.

### Miscellaneous Publications

*Consumer Information Catalog*. The catalogue in which the booklets described in this section are listed. Issued quarterly; contains useful consumer information from thirty agencies of the federal government. Topics include how to fix your car, how to save money on food, health care, energy, and many other interesting selections.

*Drug Effects Can Go Up in Smoke*, #585 (1979). Findings from the 1979 Surgeon General's report about how smoking alters the action of some commonly used medicines and drugs as well as the body's ability to use certain nutrients.

*Food and Drug Interactions*, #568H (1979). Tells how commonly used drugs affect nutritional needs, how some foods affect drug actions, and how to avoid undesirable interactions.

*Lista de Publicaciones Federales en Español para el Consumidor*, #639H (1980). A selected list of federal consumer publications in Spanish. Available in bulk quantities.

*Low-Calorie Protein Diets*, #524H (1979). Answers safety questions about low-calorie protein products for weight loss. Explains FDA labeling requirements.

*Questions and Answers about Allergies*, #595H (1977). A fact sheet for the more than 35 million Americans with allergies, about common causes, symptoms, and treatments; also tells where to write for more information.

## BOOKS AND AIDS FOR TEACHERS

Goodwin, M. T. and G. Pollen. *Creative Food Experiences for Children*. Center for Science in the Public Interest, 1755 S St., N.W., Washington, D.C. 20009, 1974. Numerous suggestions of food activities, games, and recipes for teaching children about food and nutrition. A good resource book for elementary and junior high teachers, Head Start and day-care teachers, 4-H and scout leaders, camp counselors, nutritionists, parents, and others.

*Happiness Is Fun at The Table: Eating for Children Three to Four*. University of California, Agricultural Extension Service, 960 East Street, Pittsburg, Calif. A pamphlet about feeding the 3- and 4-year-olds.

Hille, Helen M. *Food for Groups of Young Children Cared For During the Day*, Children's Bureau Publication #386, 1960. U.S. Government Printing Office, Washington, D.C. 20402.

Katz, D. and M. Goodwin. *Food: Where Nutrition, Politics and Culture Meet*. Center for Science in the Public Interest, 1755 S St., NW, Washington, D.C. 20009, n.d. A guide for high school and college teachers featuring activities to help students learn about nutrition, the importance of food choices, the role that food plays in commerce, culture, politics, ethics, and economics and about how and where food originates and is processed.

*Nutrition for Athletes: A Handbook for Coaches*. American Association for Health, Physical Education, and Recreation, 1201 Sixteenth Street, N.W., Washington, D.C. 20036, 1971.

*Nutrition Information Resources for Professionals*, NNECH publication No. 1, revised, January 1975. The National Nutrition Education Clearing House, Society for Nutrition Education, Suite 1110, 2140 Shattuck Avenue, Berkeley, Calif. 94704.

*School Lunch Action Guide*. Center for Science in the Public Interest, 1755 S St., N.W., Washington, D.C. 20009, 1976. A step-by-step action guide for improving school lunches.

*Teach Nutrition with Bulletin Boards*. Life Skills Center, Department of Home Economics, Montclair State College, Upper Montclair, N.J. 07043, n.d. Outlines basic concepts of nutrition and lists criteria for good bulletin boards.

*Teach Nutrition with Games*. Life Skills Center, Department of Home Economics, Montclair State College, Upper Montclair, N.J. 07043, n.d. Designed for both elementary and secondary levels, it gives instructions for each game, adaptation for each level, and objectives for each activity.

*Teach Nutrition with Puzzles and Activities.* Life Skills Center, Department of Home Economics, Montclair State College, Upper Montclair, N.J. 07043, n.d. Puzzles and activities designed for specific grade levels and specific nutrition concepts.

### Charts and Posters

*Chemical Cuisine,* a large chart or poster. Center for Science in the Public Interest, 1755 S St., N.W., Washington, D.C. 20009, n.d. Lists what they consider to be the degree of hazard for a large number of food additives.

*Nutrition Charts.* U.S. Department of Agriculture, Washington, D.C. 20006, 1961.

Nutrition Scoreboard Poster (18 × 24″), 1974. Center for Science in the Public Interest, 1755 S St., N.W., Washington, D.C. 20009. A brightly colored poster with nutritional ratings for over 200 foods.

### Commercial Texts, Kits, Units, and Programs*

*Be Informed on Nutrition* (Unit 17). New Readers Press, Division of Laubach Literacy International, Box 131, Syracuse, N.Y. 13210. This is remedial literacy type material for adults and teenagers written at grade levels 3.2 to 4.2. Each unit in this series provides up to 10 hours of classwork and contains exercises in reading comprehension, word study, writing, listening, and grammar skills. Single units contain about 40 pages. Teacher's guides and answer keys are provided.

The Instant Energy, Sugarcoated, Fast Food Nutrition Kit. Learning Seed Company, 145 Brentwood Drive, Palatine, Ill. 60067. Grades 7–12. The kit explains the recommendations of the Senate Select Committee on Nutrition and Human Needs. Students analyze their own diet and evaluate it in terms of sound nutrition. The kit contains two sound filmstrips with cassette narration, "Confessions of a Junk Food Junkie" and "Dietary Goals for the United States," six copies of a 32-page booklet, "Nutritional Value of Foods," a copy of Brand-name Nutrition Counter, and a silent filmstrip titled "Nutri-Test." It also contains a spirit master summary and a teaching guide in a vinyl binder.

Language and the Supermarket. Learning Seed Company, 145 Brentwood Drive, Palatine, Ill. 60067. Grades 9–12. *Language and the Supermarket: Winning the Grocery Game* was created for use in both consumer education and language arts classes and requires the skills of writing, research, information gathering, problem solving, speaking, group discussion, and critical reading. The kit contains a two-part color, sound filmstrip that explains how to play and win the supermarket game. It demonstrates how to use labels, the purpose of additives, etc. A second, silent filmstrip, the "Supermarket Survival Test," is backed by 5000 words of printed script/analysis for the teacher and a spirit master for the student. The kit also includes 144 scavenger cards to be used in local supermarkets, 35 two-page dictionary of common food additives, and a copy of *Eater's Digest,* by Michael Jacobson to be used as a reference.

Radigan, Kenneth and René Weber. *Nutrition and You.* CBS Educational Publishing, 2211 Michigan Avenue, Santa Monica, Calif. 90404, 1979. This is a nutrition education program for children in the primary grades and is divided into levels 1, 2, and 3. Each level contains lessons with objectives, materials,

---

* Presented here as examples of the types of items on the market today.

vocabulary, and procedure provided. Culminating activities are suggested, and additional fact sheets for the teacher's information are available.

White, Ruth Bennett. *You and Your Food.* Englewood Cliffs, N.J.: Prentice-Hall, 1976. This *first* foods course for grades 7–12 stresses the effect of nutrition on health, appearance, growth, development, and personality at all stages of life. It promotes intelligent consumer practices in the areas of chemical additives, fads and fallacies, organic foods, and standard labeling. A new chapter discusses careers in foods.

Also available from this publisher is the advanced foods and nutrition text for high school students entitled *Food and Your Future* by Ruth Bennett White.

## Sources for Filmstrips

Coronet, Media, 65 E. So. Water St., Chicago, Ill. 60601. Has titles such as Foods We Eat Series, etc.

Educational Activities, Inc., P.O. Box 392, Freeport, N.Y. 11520. Nutrition for Little Children (with cassettes) and others. K-up.

Eye Gate Media, Instructional Materials, 146–01 Archer Avenue, Jamaica, N.Y. 11435. Has elementary-level films such as *Basic Nutrition for Primaries, Why Do We Eat, Eating Healthy Meals Each Day, The Basic Food Groups, Eating Right Can Be Fun,* as well as others on other levels.

Learning Seed Company, 145 Brentwood Drive, Palatine, Ill. 60067. Has filmstrips and cassettes with their learning kits about nutrition for junior high through high school. They are *The Instant Energy, Sugarcoated, Fast Food Nutrition Kit* and *Language and the Supermarket.*

Marsh Film Enterprises, Inc., Box 8082, Shawnee Mission, Kan. 66208. Has among others *Food for Thought: A Matter of Choice* for upper elementary and junior high.

The Polished Apple, 3742 Seaborn Drive, Malibu, Calif. 90265. Kindergarten–grade 1 films include *The Snacking Mouse, The Polished Apple Nutrition Ed. Series, Etc.*

Ralph V. Butterworth, Inc., 25366 Cypress Ave., Hayward, Calif. 94544.

Society for Visual Education, 1345 Diversey Parkway, Chicago, Ill. 60614. Has elementary level *Four Part Series on Nutrition: Meat Foods, Milk Foods, Vegetable and Fruit Foods, Cereal and Bread Foods* suitable for lower elementary levels.

Walt Disney Educational Media Company, 500 South Buena Vista St., Burbank, Calif. 91521. Has, among others, *Winnie the Pooh, Nutrition and You: Balanced Diet—The Need for Variety, Regular Meals, Personal Choices, Meal Time—Special Time, Shopping for Good Health, Review—The Need for Healthy Habits.* Primary–elementary.

## Sources for Films

Barr Films, P.O. Box 5667, Pasadena, Calif. 91107. *All American Meal,* 11 minutes, color, 1975, grades 7–12.

Benchmark Films, Inc., P.O. Box 315, Franklin Lakes, N.J. 07417. *A Chemical Feast,* 11 minutes, color, n.d., grades 6–12.

Alfred Higgins Productions, Inc., 9100 Sunset Blvd., Los Angeles, Calif. 90069. *Eating on the Run,* 15½ minutes, color, 1975, grades 5–12.

Paramount Communications, 6912 Tujunga Ave., No. Hollywood, Calif. 91605. *The Real Talking, Singing, Action Movie about Nutrition,* 14 minutes, color, 1972, grades 4–10.

Vision Films, P.O. Box 48896, Los Angeles, Calif. 90048. *Seeing through Commercials: A Children's Guide to T.V. Advertising,* 15 minutes, color, 1976, primary–elementary.

## Films on Good Nutrition

*A Chemical Feast*
Grades 7–12, color, 11 minutes
In chef's clothes and surrounded by an array of chemicals and modified foods, comedian Marshall Ephron, in his memorable satire, merrily concocts a supermarket synthetic "lemon pie" using the ingredients listed on the label.
Benchmark Films         1976

*Eat, Drink and Be Wary*
Grades 7–12, color, 21 minutes
Shoppers, cooks, kids, and critics vent their views on our eating habits and on processed foods which now make up much of our diet. Additives, sugar content, and marketing are examined. Natural foods are advocated.
Churchill Films         1975

*Eating on the Run*
Grades 4–12, color, 16 minutes
Shows how it is possible to have a well-balanced diet even while "eating on the run." Illustrates examples of nutritious breakfasts that can be prepared in seconds and eaten "on the run." Suggestions given for properly balanced lunch and nutritious snacks.
Alfred Higgins         1975

*The Junk Food Man*
Grades 2–4, color, 11 minutes
Animated film showing why junk foods are harmful, how to spot junk foods, and explaining how the empty calories of refined sugar and white flour snacks can deaden the appetite for healthy meals.
Aims         1977

*Look Before You Eat*
Grades 8–12, color, 22 minutes
A critical examination of our eating habits and their relationship to our health, the relation of diet to disease, and the effect of advertising and promotion on our choices.
Churchill Films         1978

*Nutrition: The All-American Meal*
Grades 7–12, color, 11 minutes
Very real problems of the "quick meal" are the loss of variety in the diet and leisurely companionship at the dinner table. Good nutrition demands an understanding of all our body's needs and a real concern for good health.
Arthur Barr Films

*Real Talking, Singing, Action Movie about Nutrition*
Grades 5–10, color, 14 minutes
Kids talk to kids in their own language about the impact of food on body development, personality, and self-image. Contemporary film techniques combine with a lively cast of junior high school students to emphasize that it's up to kids themselves to decide to eat right.
Sunkist Growers         1973

*What's Good to Eat*
Grades 4–8, color, 18 minutes
A child's delight! A supermarket where he is told he can select a basket of food to eat. But all those candies, cakes, etc., aren't a wise choice. The boy learns to choose from the four food groups to get the nutrients his body needs.
Nutrition Education Series
Dairy Council of California          1969

*Food for Life*
Grades 9–12, color, 22 minutes
Starvation is not the only form of malnutrition. This film deals with the eating habits of four teenagers. Two are Americans, one is a girl and one is a boy in South America. All four are suffering from various forms of malnutrition.
Nutrition Education Series
National Dairy Council          1969

*I Feel Great*
Grades K–6, color, 10 minutes, animated
A cartoon of young farm animals that conspire with Mrs. Cow to teach Whaffor that milk is marvelous and makes animals and little boys feel great.
Whaffor Series
Gateway Productions          1954

*Nutritional Needs of Our Bodies*
Grades 4–8, color, 11 minutes
Discovers the four general groups of foods, the six nutrients which they contain, and what the nutrients supply to the body.
Coronet Instructional Media          1961

*Seeing through Commercials*
Grades 2–8, color, 15 minutes
Alerts children to the techniques and motivations behind TV commercials that are directed to them. Shows production effect, separates entertainment and promotion, and discusses nutrition claims.
Vision Films          1978

*Vitamins from Foods*
Grades 5–8, color, 21 minutes
Dr. Lind treats sailors suffering from scurvy and finds that citrus fruits cure the sick men. Fifty years later, in Java, Dr. Eijkman accidentally finds a cure for beri-beri. The student is shown how vitamins work with enzymes to break down food.
Nutrition Education Series
National Dairy Council          1968

*You and Your Food*
Grades K–6, color, 8 minutes, animated
Jiminy Cricket stresses the value of foods which are necessary to good health. Uses the analogy of the construction of an automobile to point out that proper food must be eaten for good health.
This Is You-Health Series
Walt Disney Films          1959

## PERIODICALS WITH NUTRITION INFORMATION

*Consumer Information, A Catalog of Selected Federal Publications of Consumer Interest.* Consumer Information Center, Pueblo, Col. 81009, quarterly.

*Consumer Reports.* Consumers Union of the United States, Inc., 256 Washington St., Mount Vernon, N.Y. 10550, monthly.

*Environmental Nutrition.* Newsletter. Environmental Nutrition, 15 West 84th St., Suite 1-E, New York, N.Y. 10024, bimonthly.

*Family Health.* Family Health Magazine, 149 Fifth Ave., New York, N.Y. 10010, monthly.

*Journal of Nutrition Education.* Society for Nutrition Education, 2140 Shattuck Ave., Suite 110, Berkeley, Calif. 94704, monthly.

*Nutrition Action,* Center for Science in the Public Interest, 1755 S. St., N.W., Washington, D.C. 20009, monthly.

*Nutrition Today.* Nutrition Today, Inc., 101 Ridgely Ave., P.O. Box 465, Annapolis, Md. 21404, bimonthly.

## FREE AND INEXPENSIVE
## NUTRITIONAL RESOURCE MATERIALS

Materials developed by vested interest groups such as food associations and food industries should be perused carefully and used with a certain amount of caution. A food association or industry may put special emphasis on those foods which are products of companies who fund them. The educational material may not give the full scope of information about a product, although certain limitations may be included.

When using materials developed by special interest groups, food associations and food industries, take into consideration that they have been funded by a partial source. Remember to consider whether the information promotes good eating habits, if it contains evidence for the statements or claims made, and if it presents *complete* information.

### Food Associations and Industries

Air France, P.O. Box 30729, JFK Airport Sta., Jamaica, N.Y. 11430. Free "French Recipe Booklet."

All-American Nut Co., 16901 Valley View, Cerritos, Calif. 90101. Free 16-page booklet, "An All-American Nut's Recipe Book." Send a business-size, stamped, self-addressed envelope.

American Bakers Association, 70 Pennsylvania Ave., N.W., Washington, D.C.

Ball Corporation, 345 South High Street, Muncie, Ind. 47302. Free pamphlets, recipes, booklets, and reference charts on food preservation.

Banana Bunch, 40 West 57th Street, New York, N.Y. 10019.

American Popcorn Company, Box 178, Sioux City, Iowa 51102. Free "Jolly Time Recipes for Popcorn Lovers."

Blue Goose, Inc., Education Dept., P.O. Box 46, Fullerton, Calif. 92632.

Calavo Growers of California, Box 3486, Terminal Annex, Los Angeles, Calif. 90051. Free leaflets, charts, posters, and recipes about tropical fruit such as papayas, mangoes, coconuts, kiwi fruit, limes, and avocados as well as figs, raisins, and pineapples.

Cal-Fruit, 730 Market Court, Los Angeles, Calif. 90004.

California Almond Grower's Exchange, P.O. Box 1768, Sacramento, Calif. 95808. Free "Treasury of World's Best Almond Recipes."

California Apricot Advisory Board, 1295 Boulevard Way, Suite H, Walnut Creek, Calif. 94595. Free recipe booklets, including "The Versatility of Apricots:

Exciting New Recipes for Diabetic Diets" and others. Pamphlets on history and a clever nutrition calculator of essential nutrients in canned fruits.

California Dried Fig Advisory Board, P.O. Box 709, Fresno, Calif. 93712. Free recipe leaflets, nutritional value chart, and an 11-by-14-inch poster in color.

California Frozen Vegetable Council, 27 Branan, Suite 501, San Francisco, Calif. 94107. Free advice on best cooking methods for frozen vegetables.

California Iceberg Lettuce Commission, P.O. Box 3354, Monterey, Calif. 93940. Free teacher demonstration and lesson plan, food service recipes, charts, dressing recipes, and a 23-by-33½-inch poster in color.

California Prune Advisory Board, World Trade Center, San Francisco, Calif. 94111.

California Raisin Advisory Board, P.O. Box 5335, Fresno, Calif. 93755. Free elementary school unit, experiments, games, nutritional information, recipe booklets, historical leaflet, and two colorful posters, 30 by 20 inches and 28 by 17 inches, as well as an order form for a "Selective Snackology" Teacher's Kit. This kit was developed to help teach children in grades K–3 "some very simple facts on good snacking." It includes a teacher's guide, 22-by-34-inch classroom poster, 30 miniposters to send home with students, a coloring sheet original, in-class activities for grades K–3, and no-bake recipes for healthy snacks.

Castle & Cooke Foods, 50 California Street, San Francisco, Calif. 94111.

Cereal Institute, Inc., 135 South LaSalle Street, Chicago, Ill. 50503.

Clingpeach Advisory Board of California, 1 California Street, San Francisco, Calif. 94111.

Colombo, Inc., One Danton Drive, Methuen, Mass. 01844. Free yogurt recipes made with meat, vegetables, fish, and poultry. Includes made-with-yogurt sauces, marinades, soups, and salad dressings. Send self-addressed envelope.

Dannon Milk Products, 22-11 38th Ave., Long Island City, N.Y. 11101. Free pocket calorie counter, assorted recipe leaflets, index cards, and money-saving coupons. For residents east of the Mississippi, for two booklets send your request with a stamped, self-addressed envelope for "Yogurt and You" and 25¢ for mailing and handling for the 46-page booklet "Dieting, Yogurt, and Common Sense."

Del Monte Corporation, Consumer and Educational Service, Box 3757, Room 245, San Francisco, Calif. 94119.

Fleischmann's Margarine, P.O. Box 1-K, Elm City, N.C. 27898. Free 38-page brochure, "Low Sodium Diets Can Be Delicious," which contains 100 recipes.

Fleischmann's Yeast, P.O. Box 509, Dept. MW, Madison Square Sta., New York, N.Y. 10010. Free booklet, "The Young Cook's Bake a Bread Book," which teaches how to bake fresh bread through a series of cartoons and rhymes. Send a stamped, self-addressed, long envelope.

Florida Citrus Commission, Box 148, Lakeland, Fla. 33802.

Green Giant Company, Home Services, Le Sueur, Minn. 56058.

Grocery Manufacturers of America, 1424 K Street, NW, Washington, D.C. 20009.

Growers' Peanut Food Promotions, P.O. Box 1709, Rocky Mount, N.C. 27801. Free nutritional and historical information, recipes, and teaching topics and activities suggestions. Also two posters, one of them 16¾ by 24¼ inches.

Kansas Wheat Commission, 1021 N. Main, Hutchinson, Kansas 67501. Free nutritional information, diabetic information, posters, recipes, sample wheat bread in a plastic bubble, whole wheat kernels, a bowl scraper, recipes, weight-loss information, and more.

Kellogg Company, Department of Home Economics Services, Battle Creek, Mich. 49016.

Kraft Foods, Dept. E.P.O., Box 4611, Chicago, Ill. 60677.

La Choy Oriental Recipes, P.O. Box 47842, Dallas, Texas 75247. The recipe booklet featuring 40 recipes, "The Wonderful World of Oriental Cookery," requires 50¢ for mailing and handling.

Lamb Education Center, 200 Clayton St., Denver, Colo. 80206. Free recipe book, "Economy Lamb Cut Recipes."

Lawry's Foods, Inc., General Offices, 568 San Fernando Road, Los Angeles, Calif. 90065.

Lender's Bagel Bakery, P.O. Box 7705, Orange, Conn. 96477. Free recipe ideas using bagels. Send a stamped, self-addressed envelope.

Libby, McNeill & Libby, Inc., 200 South Michigan Avenue, Chicago, Ill. 60604. Free recipe leaflets, consumer tips booklet, information sheets, and order list of educational materials in bulk.

Lipton Kitchens, Dept. PD, T. J. Lipton, 800 Sylvan Ave., Englewood Cliffs, N.J. 07632. Free copy of 34 recipes using noodles entitled "Noodle Recipes."

Louisiana Sweet Potato Commission, P.O. Box 113, Opelousas, La. 70570.

Mazola Corn Oil or Best Foods, Box 307, Coventry, Conn. 96238. Free booklets "A Diet for Today" outlines moderate to low-cholesterol menus and features 3( recipes for dishes included in the menus; write to Dept. DT-1001. For the othei booklet, "Eating Well," write to Dept. EW-1001. Tells about how good nutrition in the young years safeguards your health as you grow older and gives nutrition facts. Best Foods' free booklet "Good Recipes to Brighten the Allergy Diet" contains dessert recipes that contain no wheat, eggs, or milk. Available through Dept. GRA-1001. Write to Dept. LL-1001 for a list of other free materials.

Meals of Millions, P.O. Box 680, Santa Monica, Calif. 90496. Free are 6 meatless recipes such as spinach casserole, sweet and sour soybeans, ratatouille Monterey, and other meatless meals to nourish your family without robbing your bank balance.

Metropolitan Life Insurance Co., Health and Welfare Division, 1 Madison Avenue, New York, N.Y. 10010.

NABC, P.O. Box 38, Tuckahoe, N.J. 08250. Free booklet on easy ways to prepare blueberry recipes using fresh, frozen, or canned blueberries with tips for efficient freezing and storage; 15-cent handling charge at time of publication.

Nabisco Company, 525 Park Avenue, New York, N.Y. 10022. Has radio scripts available, among other things.

National Dairy Council, 6300 N. River Road, Rosemont, Ill. 60018.

National Livestock and Meat Board, Nutrition Research Department, 444 N. Michigan Avenue, Chicago, Ill. 60611.

New England Fish Co., Pier 89, Seattle, Wash. 98119. Free recipe booklet, "Quick and Easy Ways with Salmon," tells how to make high-calcium, high-protein dishes using canned salmon.

New Zealand Meat Producers Board, 800 Third Avenue, New York, N.Y. 10022. Free full-color 24-page booklet of recipes using New Zealand lamb.

North Carolina Yam Commission, P.O. Box 12005, Raleigh, N.C. 27605.

Nutrition Information Service, Consumer Service Department, Best Foods, Division of CPC International, International Plaza, Englewood Cliffs, N.J. 07632.

Oregon, Washington and California Pear Bureau, 601 Woodlark Building, Dept. F, Portland, Ore. 97205.

Peanut Association, Inc., 342 Madison Avenue, New York, N.Y. 10017.

Pet Incorporated, 400 South Fourth Street, St. Louis, Mo. 63106. Free recipe booklets, leaflets, and cards.

Pillsbury Company, Box 60-090, Minneapolis, Minn. 55460. Games, booklets, and posters available for a nominal fee.

Poultry and Egg National Board, 18 South Michigan Avenue, Chicago, Ill. 60603.

Potato Board, 1385 S. Colorado Blvd. Denver, Colo. 80222.

Quaker Oats Company, Merchandise Mart, Chicago, Ill. 60654.

Rice Council, P.O. Box 22802, Houston, Texas 77027. Free booklets including "Rice . . . Low Calorie Menus and Recipes," "Great Dinners for Six . . . on a Budget," "Southern Rice Recipes," and "Rice Salads."

Rock Lobster, Room 3500, 450 Seventh Avenue, New York, N.Y. 10001.

Roquefort Association, Inc., 41 East 42nd Street, New York, N.Y. 10017. Free brochure about the cheese as well as a 38-page recipe booklet. This cheese is still made exclusively of sheeps' milk.

Skippy, Dept. USP-1001, Box 307, Coventry, Conn. 06238. A free illustrated story booklet, "The Unusual Story of the Peanut," takes the reader from the peanut on the vine through history and finally to peanut butter at the Skippy plant.

Spanish Olive Oil Institute, 666 Fifth Avenue, New York, N.Y. 10019. A booklet, "Cooking the Natural Way with Spanish Olive Oil" contains 48 recipes using ingredients that contain few or no preservatives; 25¢ for mailing and handling.

Standard Brands Education Service, P.O. Box 2695, Grand Central Station, New York, N.Y. 10017.

Standard Oil Co. of California, 16 Spear Street, San Francisco, Calif. 94105.

Stokely–Van Camp, Inc., Home Economics Dept., 491 N. Meridian Street, Indianapolis, Ind. 46206. Free pamphlets, recipe booklets, and posters as well as a sheet on cooking canned and frozen vegetables. (Also available for $1.00 is a teaching guide to help high school home economics students learn the value and variety of nutritious meal-planning ideas with fruits and vegetables. This kit, "Enjoying Vegetables," includes six spirit duplicating masters, one transparency, and a file folder with a complete teacher's guide.)

Sunkist Growers, P.O. Box 2706, Terminal Annex, Los Angeles, Calif. 90054. Puppets, games, and other materials available.

Swift and Company, 1919 Swift Drive, Oak Brook, Ill. 60521.

Switzerland Cheese Association, 444 Madison Ave., New York, N.Y. 10022. Free booklet, "Fat in Cheese," gives you fat facts—the percentage of fat in cheeses, etc.

United Fresh Fruit and Vegetable Association, Instructor's Educational Service, Box 510, Daneville, New York, N.Y. 14437.

Table Grape Commission of California, P.O. Box 5498, Fresno, Calif. 93755.

Vitamin Information Service, Hoffman-LaRoche Ins., Nutley, N.J. 07110. Free booklet, "Food Labels: The Guide to Better Nutrition."

Washington Apple Commission, P.O. Box 18, Wenatchee, Wash. 98801. Free nutritional information and recipe leaflets and the "Apple Notebook," a specially designed leaflet for photocopy reproduction that contains nutritional, historical, purchasing, care and storage information as well as use and preparation tips.

Weight Watchers International, 800 Community Dr., Manhasset, N.Y. 11030. Free brochure, "Weight Control and You," is available.

Wheat Flour Institute, 309 W. Jackson Blvd., Chicago, Ill. 60606.

## Special Interest Groups, Governmental and Other Agencies

American Association for Health, Physical Education and Recreation, 1201 16th Street, N.W., Washington, D.C. 20036.

Action for Children's Television, 46 Austin Street, Newtonville, Mass. 02160.

American Dental Association, 211 E. Chicago Ave., Chicago, Ill. 60611.

American Dietetics Association, 620 N. Michigan, Chicago, Ill. 60611.

American Heart Association, 44 East 23rd Street, New York, N.Y. 10010. Free booklets from your local Heart Association include "The Way to a Man's Heart" (51-018-A), "Recipes for Fat-controlled Low Cholesterol Meals" (50-020-B), and "A Guide to Weight Reduction" (50-034-A).

American Home Economics Association, 2010 Massachusetts Ave., N.W., Washington, D.C. 20036.

American Institute of Nutrition, 9650 Rockville Place, Bethesda, Md. 20014.

American Medical Association, 535 N. Dearborn Street, Chicago, Ill. 60610.

American National Red Cross, Food and Nutrition Consultant, 17th Street NW, between D and E Streets, National Headquarters, Washington, D.C. 20006.

American School Food Service Association, 4101 East Iliff Ave., Denver, Colo. 80222.

California State Department of Education, Nutrition Education and Training Program, 721 Capitol Mall, Sacramento, Calif. 95814.

Center for Science in the Public Interest, 1779 Church Street, Washington, D.C. 20036.

Committee on Children's Television Inc., 1511 Masonic Ave., San Francisco, Calif. 94117.

Executive Health, Pickfair Building, Rancho Santa Fe, Calif. 92067.

Food and Drug Administration, Consumer Information, Public Documents Distribution Center, Pueblo, Colo., 81009.

Food and Nutrition Board, National Research Council, 2101 Constitution Ave., Washington, D.C. 20418.

Good Vend Campaign, 1757 S. Street, N.W., Washington, D.C. 20009. Organization for nutritious vended food.

National Foundation March of Dimes, Birth Defects Foundation, 1275 Mamaroneck Avenue, White Plains, N.Y. 10605. Free materials available on nutrition during pregnancy.

Nutrition Today Society, 1500 Eckington Place, N.E., Washington, D.C. 20002.

Society for Nutrition Education, 2140 Shattuck Ave., Suite 110, Berkeley, Calif. 94704.

Superintendent of Documents, Government Printing Office, Washington, D.C. 20402.

USDA, Jefferson Drive between 12th and 14th Streets, SW, Washington, D.C. 20250. See also your County Cooperative Extension Service.

United States Department of H.E.W., FDS, 5600 Fisher Lane, Rockville, Md. 20852.

United States Environmental Protection Agency, Washington, D.C. 20460.

United States Committee for UNICEF, 331 E. 38th Street, New York, N.Y. 10016.

## ADDITIONAL SOURCES OF
## NUTRITION INFORMATION

For reliable general information about nutrition contact your city, county or state health department's nutritionist or the nutritionist at the local gas or electric company. For queries about special diet problems, contact a registered dietitian or nutritionist at your local or state volunteer health organization such as the heart or diabetes association, at your local or state public health department, or at your local hospital or clinic.

# Index

# About the Author

Dr. Lendon Smith has been practicing pediatrics since 1951. During the past seven years he has particularly emphasized nutritional counseling for parents. Dr. Smith is former Clinical Professor of Pediatrics at the University of Oregon Medical School and a member of the American Academy of Pediatrics. He became a favorite of television viewers for his television show *The Children's Doctor*—also the title of his first book—and won an Emmy for his television documentary *My Mom's Having a Baby*. Dr. Smith is a frequent guest on the major network television shows and is the author of the best-selling *Improving Your Child's Behavior Chemistry* and *Feed Your Kids Right*.